This interdisciplinary account provides an integrated and practical guide to the management and treatment of burns. Experts from all the major disciplines involved in critical care have focused their attention on specific problems and areas of treatment involved in the care of burned patients. Although it is essentially a practical guide to the management of thermal injury, with explicit recommendations for courses of treatment, it also provides explanatory background information on the manifestations and clinical consequences of this common source of injury.

CRITICAL CARE OF THE BURNED PATIENT

CRITICAL CARE OF THE BURNED PATIENT

Edited by

LINDSEY T.A. RYLAH

Director of Critical Care, Regional Burns Unit,
St Andrew's Hospital, Billericay, Essex, UK

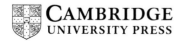

CAMBRIDGE
UNIVERSITY PRESS

Published by the Press Syndicate of the University of Cambridge
The Pitt Building, Trumpington Street, Cambridge CB2 1RP
40 West 20th Street, New York, NY 10011-4211, USA
10 Stamford Road, Oakleigh, Victoria 3166, Australia

First published 1992

Printed in Great Britain by Redwood Press Limited, Melksham, Wiltshire

A catalogue record for this book is available from the British Library

Library of Congress cataloguing in publication data

Critical care of the burned patient / edited by Lindsey T.A. Rylah.
    p.   cm.
Includes index.
ISBN 0-521-39495-3 (hardback)
1. Burns and scalds – Treatment.   2. Critical care medicine.
I. Rylah, Lindsey T.A.
[DNLM: 1. Burns – therapy.   2. Critical Care.   WO 704 C934]
RD96.4.C77   1992
617.1′ 106 – dc20
DNLM/DLC
for Library of Congress   92-7867 CIP

ISBN 0 521 39495 3 hardback

RD96.4
C 77
1992

To Barbara,
Barnaby, Freddie,
Osgar, and Joshua

Contents

ix

Contributors

Ahrenholz, D.H.
St Paul-Ramsey Medical Center
640 Jackson Street, St. Paul, Minnesota 55101, USA

Bessey, P.Q.
Barnes Hospital
Barnes Hospital Plaza, St Louis, Missouri 63110, USA

Bunsell, R.
Regional Burns Unit
Stoke Mandeville Hospital, Mandeville Road, Aylesbury, Bucks. HP21 8AL,
UK

Clark, W.R.
Associate Professor of Surgery, State University of New York Health Science
Center
Syracuse University, New York, USA

Edbrooke, D.
Royal Hallamshire Hospital
Glossop Road, Sheffield S10 2JF, UK

Finkelstein, J.L.
New York Hospital
Cornell Medical Center, 525E 68th Street, Manhattan, New York 10021, USA

Goodwin, C.W.
New York Hospital
Cornell Medical Center, 525E 68th Street, Manhattan, New York 10021, USA

Hunt, J.
Parkland Memorial Hospital
Dallas, Texas 75235, USA

John, R.E.
Royal Hallamshire Hospital
Glossop Road, Sheffield S10 2JF, UK

Kagan, R.J.
University of Cincinnati Medical Center
Department of Surgery, 231 Bethesda Avenue, Cincinnati, Ohio 45267-0558,
USA

Madden, M.R.
New York Hospital
Cornell Medical Center, 525E 68th Street, Manhattan, New York 10021, USA

Marano, M.A.
New York Hospital
Cornell Medical Center, 525E 68th Street, Manhattan, New York 10021, USA

Monafo, W.
Department of Surgery
Washington University School of Medicine, Box 8109, 4960 Audobon,
St. Louis, Missouri 63110, USA

Murray, R.J.
Royal Hallamshire Hospital
Glossop Road, Sheffield S10 2JF, UK

Purdue, G.F.
Parkland Memorial Hospital
Dallas, Texas 75235, USA

Rylah, L.T.A.
St Andrew's Hospital
Stock Road, Billericay, Essex CM12 0BH, UK

Solem, L.D.
St Paul-Ramsey Medical Center
640 Jackson Street, St Paul, Minnesota 55101, USA

Underwood, S.M.
Anaesthetics Department
Bristol Royal Infirmary, Marlborough Street, Bristol BS2 8HW, UK

Ward, G.
University of Miami
Jackson Memorial Hospital, 1611 N.W. 12th Avenue, Miami, Florida 33136,
USA

Warden, G.D.
Shriners Hospital for Crippled Children
Burns Institute, 202 Goodman Street, Cincinnati, Ohio 45219, USA

Williams, J.B.
St Paul-Ramsey Medical Center
640 Jackson Street, St Paul, Minnesota 55101, USA

Wilmshurst, A.D.
Odstock Hospital
Salisbury, Wilts. SP2 8BJ, UK

Preface

'What is needed is a practical guide to burn treatment.' This is a statement often made by residents. Many books have been written, but most are written in the style of a collection of review articles. This book has been compiled with the aim of being pragmatic and answering the question: 'What should I do?' If the chapter does not answer this question, then it will point the questioner in the right direction to obtain his own answer. Each chapter can be read on its own and thus there are occasional overlaps and repetitions when the book is read as a whole.

The book is aimed at residents in surgery, anaesthesia and intensive care but will be useful to all, both medical and nursing, who may come across burns and be required to treat them.

Lindsey Rylah

Acknowledgements

—

I would like to thank all the staff of the NE Thames Regional Burns Unit, both nursing and medical, who have helped and encouraged me in the production of this book. Special thanks must go to Anne Rider who typed the manuscript as a labour of love for the Unit.

1

Pathophysiology of burn shock

W.W. MONAFO, P.Q. BESSEY

Introduction

One of the major advances in acute burn care of this century is the appreciation of the importance and adoption of the practice of prompt and aggressive fluid resuscitation of the burn victim. Thirty years ago, the majority of patients with extensive burns died from burn shock within the first week following their injuries. Today, however, early death can usually be prevented in previously healthy individuals and is seen only in those with near total body surface burns or in those of advanced age or with major concurrent chronic disease.

There have been advances in a variety of other areas which have also contributed to improved outcome from major burns. These include improved emergency medical services and the general availability of adequately trained teams to provide life-saving treatment both at the scene and during rapid ground or air transport; the prompt referral of patients with major burn injuries to specialized burn centres where teams of experienced and knowledgeable professionals direct management; major advances in cardiopulmonary, respiratory and metabolic monitoring and supportive care and in nutrition; and finally, improved wound management techniques.

After a brief historical perspective, the major local and systemic pathophysiological phenomena which will follow burn injury will be reviewed.

Historical perspective

To appreciate the impact fluid resuscitation has had on burn victims, it is useful to review the natural history of a major burn without treatment.

Since this is rarely observed today, a description written by the Austrian dermatologist, W.K. Kaposi (1837–1902) is quoted:

'Let us take an average case, such as is presented when the clothing of a person has been ignited by burning alcohol, petroleum, gas, etc, the flame, as usual, immediately striking upward so as to affect largely the face and arms. Let us assume, furthermore, that the fire has been smothered in from one to three minutes by persons present. Ordinarily, the following picture is presented one or two hours after the catastrophe. The hair over the face and head is singed; burns are present over the hands and forearms, here and there about the upper arms, the face, the neck and clavicular region, the nucha, the upper dorsal region, and the lower extremities. At points where the clothes fit closely or bands constrict, the skin is least injured by a rapid flame, as for instance under the corset, around the waist, and under the garters.

The greater portion of the injury is of first and second degree; only limited areas about the face, the chest, generally also the back, exhibit brown carbonization, or a white eschar of the epidermis which has been detached by the exudation or mechanically by attempts to quench the fire. Hence, burn of the third degree is either lacking or present to a very limited extent.

The course, then, is the following: the patient, who during and immediately after the accident was excited to the highest degree and acted almost insanely, screaming and lamenting, becomes quiet as soon as the injuries are skilfully dressed. He bears the burning sensations without complaint or at most emits faint groans or whines. Otherwise, he is entirely rational and in possession of his mental powers.

On being questioned, he relates the details of the accident and gives the minutest particulars about everything. As a rule, he has not urinated since. On introducing the catheter, there is generally not a trace of urine; occasionally, a few drops are obtained which are albuminous or, more rarely, bloody. After five or six hours, we notice from time to time yawning and deep sighs; the eyelids are kept closed. On being addressed, the patient looks up and gives correct answers, but a certain apathy is unmistakably present. Then there will be often deep inspiration and eructations or hiccough. This is a bad sign.

Soon there will be vomiting of remnants of food, bilious fluid, or rarely, even blood. Hebra has stated that on opening different veins he failed to obtain a stream of blood. My own venesections produced a vigorous flow of blood. Now there rapidly follow restlessness, confusion, jactitation, clonic convulsions, opisthotonos, and absolute insensibility. Noisy delirium gives place to quiet sopor, or the latter immediately follows the former apathy. In the course of these symptoms, with rapid, shallow respiration and frequent, vanishing pulse, in the midst of a screaming and noisy spell, or else in quiet sopor, death ensues in the course of eighteen to twenty-four or forty-eight hours. Sometimes this is preceded by haemorrhages from the stomach and bladder. I have seen very few patients recover in whom ischuria was present or singultus and vomiting occurred.'

Unfortunately, the similarities between shock that develops in acutely burned patients and that which occurs in other illnesses, in which plasma and extracellular fluid volumes are depleted, were not recognized at the time of Kaposi's description. Several decades earlier, O'Shaugnessy had made pioneering observations that led to the recognition of the restorative effects of intravenous sodium salt solutions in hypovolaemic circulatory shock. He found that the blood of patients with acute Asiatic cholera had 'lost a large proportion of its water' and as well 'a great proportion of its neutral saline ingredients' (Lancet i:1831). Thomas Latta in London was aware of O'Shaugnessy's report, and he was the first to administer intravenous saline solution to patients with florid hypovolaemic shock. The cause of fluid loss in these patients was cholera, and Latta saw dramatic improvement. In one woman of 50, he boldly administered 10 litres in 12 hours . . . 'when reaction was completely re-established and in 48 hours she smoked her pipe free from distemper'.

In the early 1900s, scattered clinical reports of the beneficial effects of saline in burn shock began to appear, such as the paper by the American psychiatrist, Sneve in 1905.[1] However, it was many years later in the mid–20th century before the importance of volume resuscitation in shock following trauma in general was recognized[2,3] and before the magnitude of the fluid shifts which invariably attend burns was fully appreciated.[4-7]

Shortly following World War II, blood banking was widely introduced. Plasma and other blood fractions and albumin became available. Early policies for the use of whole blood in treating haemorrhagic shock[8] were soon followed by recommendations that plasma or human serum albumin should comprise major components of the fluid resuscitation in acutely burned patients.[4-7] Evidence had accumulated that plasma volume was regularly decreased within a few hours after major burn injury and that the fluid which formed in the vicinity of the wound and in the wound blisters was 'plasma-like'.[2] It therefore seemed appropriate to give what had been lost. The fluid therapy prescriptions of this era ('budgets' or 'formulae' as they were called)[6,7,9,10] included water, salt, and albumin or plasma. These were the forerunners of present-day recommendations and practice.

During the past 30 years sodium salt solutions have been established as the most important and essential component of fluid therapy for burn shock. The original burn 'formulae' carried an arbitrary volume limit (the burn area was not to be calculated at more than 50% TBSA, irrespective of its actual size) because of the concern that acute heart failure from volume overload would occur. However, this restriction has since been discarded, as has the recommendation that electrolyte-free, 5% glucose and water be given for 'metabolic needs'. Indeed, impressive fluid volumes are now known to be necessary to resuscitate some patients successfully. [11–13] Furthermore, the role, timing, and potential hazards of adjuvant therapy with fluids containing macromolecular solutes such as human serum albumin, dextran, hydroxyethyl starch, etc (the so-called 'colloids') is now better appreciated.[14,15]

Pathophysiology

The development of burn shock is determined by events which occur in the burn wound. The 'burn' injury itself results in coagulation necrosis of a certain mass of tissue which has both breadth and depth; that is surface area and depth or degree. The mass of cells between this coagulum and normal tissue comprise a three-dimensional zone of injury, and this is an important component of the burn wound. It is here that oedema rapidly accumulates. Depending on the local severity of the burn, the true 'wound' may extend into the subcutaneous tissues or even into the muscle or deep soft tissues, irrespective of the ultimate depth of skin loss. Unfortunately, many experimental studies of fluid flux in burn wounds are flawed because they either presume that vascular injury is confined to the skin (i.e. the dermis) or ignore examination of the fluid fluxes in the subjacent tissues even though these are often so large that the oedema is grossly visible.[16]

If the wound volume is sufficiently large (e.g. a burn whose surface dimensions include 15–20% or more of the total body surface area (TBSA) in a previously healthy adult, the oedema volume sequestered will be sufficiently large that systemic signs of hypovolaemia will sooner or later appear during the succeeding 24 hours. If the burn area is of modest size, compensatory physiological responses may delay or even occasionally prevent the appearance of overt shock. Fluid therapy in many, if not most, instances is instituted prior to the appearance of overt shock: the therapy is therefore actually preventative or prophylactic in nature. On the other hand, overt shock may be present within minutes post-injury in patients with massive burns.

Anatomical correlates

Microvascular injury and interstitial oedema are consistent findings in thermally injured soft tissue. Gaps appear early between endothelial

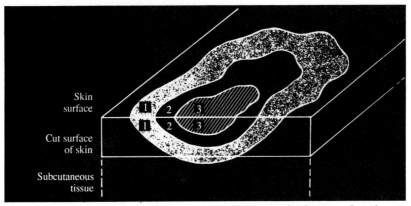

Fig. 1.1. Zones of injury. 1: zone of hyperaemia; 2: zone of stasis; 3: zone of necrosis.

cells. The venular endothelium is probably the most susceptible, but as injury severity increases, inter-endothelial gaps become visible in capillaries and arterioles as well.[17] Large molecules which are normally mainly retained within exchange vessels (such as Evans blue, which binds to circulating albumin) readily extravasate through the abnormal gaps into the extravascular tissues when they are injected shortly after injury.[4,5,18,19] To a more limited extent, red cells also extravasate. As the endothelial injury matures, there is platelet aggregation on the injured endothelium; this eventuates in frank microthrombosis, which may progressively extend proximally into larger distributive vessels. In zones of full thickness injury, there is confluent dermal vascular thrombosis. Oedema formation in areas where the circulation has been obliterated is relatively minimal, but becomes progressively more pronounced toward the periphery of the injury, where blood still circulates, if sluggishly, through the injured but still patent exchange vasculature (Fig. 1.1).

Loss of microvascular integrity: time course of oedema formation

The loss of microvascular integrity in thermally injured tissues is presently thought to be mediated by vasoactive and/or toxic agents released by the injured tissues which act in concert to increase fluid flux into the interstitium. Bradykinin, histamine, prostaglandins, oxygen and hydroxyl free radicals and leukotrienes have all been implicated, but detailed knowledge of the events which occur at the cellular or molecular level is lacking. To date, there is no clinically applicable means of inhibiting or reversing burn oedema by systemically or topically administering pharmacological inhibitors of these substances in the early post-injury period; although in scalded rodents, pre-treatment with the histamine H₂ blocker cimetidine may decrease oedema formation.[20]

Both experimentally and clinically, oedema formation is most rapid during the first few hours post-injury. About 80% of the total oedema is present within 4 to 6 hours.[13,21] Clinically, oedema accumulation continues for a variable period, up to 24 or 36 hours, after which, for reasons that are unknown, spontaneous partial resorption begins; this is associated with a concomitant increase in plasma volume and a more or less (especially in the elderly) abrupt decrease in fluid therapy requirements.

Experimentally, oedema formation has been studied indirectly by cannulation of lymphatic vessels draining burned or scalded skin and measuring the rate of wound lymph flow and its protein content.[19,21] Within minutes, there is a marked increase in flow, followed by a slower but protracted rise. The lymph is protein rich. In the elegant studies of Parker *et al.*, lymph total protein content increased four-fold despite a concomitant five-fold increase in total lymph flow, indicating that a dramatic rise in microvascular permeability had occurred.[21] The loss of the normal sieving effect of the microvasculature appeared to be the result of an increase in microvascular filtration through large (400 Å) pores, which accounted for about 50% of macromolecular sieving in the post-burn period, compared to only 13% prior to injury. These investigators also found that blood flow increased to the burn wound and that capillary pressure rose, presumably as the result of a decrease in pre-capillary resistance. They concluded that the rate of oedema formation could not be accounted for by an increase in capillary permeability alone and that the capillary pressure increase was responsible for approximately one-half of the increased rate of fluid flux. These findings would explain in part the failure of pharmacological blockade of the mediators mentioned above to minimize oedema formation. Others have suggested that osmotically active molecules are released from injured cells in the wound which attract fluid (oedema) until osmotic equilibrium is achieved.[22]

Sodium content of oedema fluid

Oedema fluid obtained either directly from surface blisters or the sub-escharotic space or as a supernatant of centrifuged wound tissue homogenates has an electrolyte content closely resembling that of plasma. However, when the net gains in sodium and water content of the entire wound (injury zone) are determined, the sodium content of the accumulated oedema is found to be moderately hypertonic with respect to the concentration of sodium in the plasma and extracellular fluid. Phenomena which may account for this include:

1. the transfer of sodium into thermally injured or killed cells in exchange for potassium;
2. a similar transfer of sodium into cells injured as a result of cell membrane ischaemia due to inadequate or delayed resuscitation;[23]
3. adsorption of sodium ions on thermally injured collagen.[24–26]

The apparent disproportionate sequestration of sodium into injured tissue emphasizes the importance of the sodium ion in resuscitation and suggests that hypertonic sodium salt solutions might be of special benefit.

Fluid therapy increases oedema

In the absence of fluid therapy, spontaneous oedema accumulation in the burn wound is greater per unit wound weight in small burns than in extensive burns for injuries of identical local severity which differ only in their surface area.[16] The explanation appears to be that the available pool of extracellular fluid from which the oedema is extracted is finite. Small surface area wounds will accumulate near-maximal oedema spontaneously, while extensive wounds will swell to an identical extent only after fluid therapy. During the acute phase of burn shock, fluid resuscitation refills the depleted extracellular fluid reservoir, restores and maintains the circulation to the wound, and thereby promotes extravascular water flux.

Although fluid therapy is necessary in order to prevent death from shock, it unavoidably increases local oedema formation. Furthermore, the hypo-proteinaemia which typically develops may promote oedema formation in non-burned tissues.[27] Thus, the fluid volume ultimately required may be quite large, amounting to 20–30% or more of the body weight within the first 24 hours in severe injuries. Close clinical monitoring is necessary to avoid under treatment on the one hand and unnecessary over-infusion of resuscitation fluids on the other. The non-cardiopulmonary effects of this oedema accumulation are unclear, but since the circulation in the wound is already impaired as the result of endothelial injury and microvascular thrombosis, additional therapy related oedema and elevated tissue pressure might further compromise wound blood flow, perpetuating ischaemia and resulting in additional cellular injury.[28]

Clinical features of burn shock

The clinical findings in established burn shock are no different from those of other forms of hypovolaemic shock. The patients are restless, thirsty, perhaps disorientated, or in advanced cases, near-comatose. They have hypotension, tachycardia, tachypnoea and may have cyanosis of unburned skin. But if cutaneous injury is the sole problem, overt shock will not ordinarily be present until several hours or more have elapsed, even in patients with extensive burns.

The initial presence or rapid development of an impaired mental state or of hypotension should suggest that other problems may exist in addition to the cutaneous injuries. The most frequent associated problem in patients with flame burns is, of course, inhalation injury which is often accompanied by carbon monoxide intoxication. However, head injury (focal neurological signs, impaired mentation), spinal cord injury (resistant hypotension, paresis), or abdominal and chest injuries (hypotension, respiratory distress or abnormal physical examination) must also be considered and appropriate diagnostic and therapeutic procedures instituted.

Typically, overt hypotension will not be present initially, and the patient will be able to relate the circumstance of the injury, as in the case described by Kaposi. Furthermore, associated inhalation injury, unless it is very severe, may not be manifested initially by stridor, hoarseness, other signs of impending airway obstruction or by rales, wheezes or rhonchi. Tachycardia, thirst, haemoconcentration and oliguria are the usual presenting features. They indicate that haemodynamic decompensation will shortly occur unless adequate fluid therapy is instituted. As in all forms of trauma, a careful history and a complete physical examination must be performed. It is particularly important to exclude other associated injuries when a fall, vehicular crash or an explosion have occurred.

Laboratory abnormalities

An arterial blood sample must be obtained initially for measurement of blood gases and pH, and sufficient venous blood for the following determinations: complete blood count; electrolytes; osmolality; blood

group; total protein and albumin; glucose; calcium. In babies, microana-
lytical methods must be used to avoid significant blood loss due to the
necessity of repetitive determinations.

The haemoglobin and haematocrit are both elevated as a result of
plasma volume loss and usually continue to rise moderately even in the
face of a satisfactory clinical response to fluid therapy during the first 12
hours or more of treatment. Provided that the response to therapy is
satisfactory as noted by the criteria below, haemoconcentration need not
be a cause of concern, and specific treatment of it (such as increasing the
rate of fluid administration) is unnecessary. After 24–36 hours, the
haemoglobin and haematocrit will typically begin to fall rapidly, events
which coincide with a decreased fluid therapy requirement and signify
that the phase of extravascular fluid flux is over and that reconstitution of
the functional extracellular fluid and plasma spaces has commenced.
During the subsequent 48–72 hours, there is ordinarily a continued rapid
fall in the haemoglobin and haematocrit to the extent that, in large burns,
blood transfusion may be necessary within the first week in order to
maintain the haemoglobin and haematocrit at reasonable (>30 haematocrit) levels to insure that blood oxygen carriage is adequate.

The white blood count is elevated initially, and in children the rise may
be striking ('leukemoid' reaction). A progressive leucopaenia, which
may be accentuated by topical therapy with silver sulphadiazine (described elsewhere) becomes evident after 72–96 hours in the post-
resuscitative phase. The differential white blood count initially shows a
shift to the left. The platelet count initially is normal or moderately
elevated. The prothrombin and partial thromboplastin times are not
typically abnormal.

If the initial (first few hours) haemoglobin and haematocrit values are
low, and a pre-existent cause of anaemia is not elicited historically, the
presence of an occult acute or chronic bleeding source must be considered.

Urine present initially at the time of catheterization is measured and
then discarded; a complete examination of urine which subsequently
appears is performed, including the osmolality and microscopic examination of the spun sediment. The urine is typically concentrated, strongly
acidic and may contain appreciable amounts of glucose, but little sodium.

If the urine is grossly red or rusty and haematuria is not verified
microscopically, haemochromagens (haemoglobin, myoglobin) are
presumptively present and their concentration must be quantitated
biochemically. Pigmenturia is characteristic in high-voltage electrical

burns and is also present in some extensive, deep, full thickness thermal injuries which involve muscle.

The potassium level is typically elevated or high normal initially due to the release of potassium from injured cells. Those receiving diuretics previously may evidence hypokalaemia severe enough to warrant replacement therapy; this must be given cautiously after fluid therapy has been initiated and the desired level of urine output achieved for several hours. Metabolic acidosis, which is roughly proportionate to injury severity is characteristic. The plasma CO_2 content is decreased. The chloride is normal or moderately elevated. The blood gases reflect compensation for the metabolic acidosis, the arterial pH being normal or low. The arterial lactate is not sharply elevated unless overt shock or an untreated muscle compartment syndrome is present, and an anion gap of significance (>14 mEq) should not be present. Plasma osmolality should be normal, although alcohol (most commonly) or other foreign substances in the blood may elevate it. The calcium is moderately depressed in proportion to the hypoalbuminaemia associated with injury and resuscitation. The plasma sodium is normal initially in the absence of previous diuretic therapy, although if lactated Ringer's, which is hypotonic with respect to sodium, has been administered in the field in appreciable volume, plasma sodium will tend to approach 130 mEq/l.

Cardiovascular changes

Cardiac output falls promptly (within minutes) after extensive burns, both clinically and experimentally. As the fall in cardiac output appreciably precedes a major fall in plasma volume (which appears subsequently), a circulating myocardial depressant factor (presumably released from the burn wound) has been postulated to play a role in the early development of burn shock. [29,30] Direct evidence of the presence of such a myocardial depressant factor is lacking. However, a recent study by Horton and her colleagues documented impairment of myocardial contractile function in isolated perfused hearts following experimental thermal injury. [31] This effect was in part age related, in that hearts of older animals were impaired to a greater extent than those of young ones, and it was not eliminated by adequate fluid resuscitation.

As fluid therapy is administered, cardiac output progressively returns to normal or above by 24–36 hours, following which it continues to rise progressively during the subsequent 4–7 days as the 'flow' phase of hypermetabolism becomes established.

Moderate tachycardia is typically present, especially in younger patients. In adults, the range is usually 100–130 per minute in the face of adequate resuscitation. Arterial blood pressure should remain within the normal or pre-injury range in uncomplicated cases.

The central venous pressure and the capillary wedge pressure are both low normal and may approach zero, even in the presence of a satisfactory response to resuscitation. Experience has shown that in those patients in whom a pulmonary artery catheter is in place during the resuscitative phase, attempts to elevate cardiac filling pressures to the normal range are unwise, as this leads to the administration of far larger fluid volumes than would otherwise be necessary. Pulmonary artery catheters are not routinely necessary for proper management during the shock phase. Their use must be restricted to patients with impaired cardiac response (usually elderly) or to patients who fail to respond appropriately to initial fluid resuscitation. Experience has shown that pulmonary artery catheters are required for the treatment of acute burn shock in only about 5–10% of patients.

As noted already, a progressive decline in plasma volume occurs for a variable period (usually 12–18 hours) even during a clinically adequate response to therapy; the fluid therapy presumably blunts the rate and extent of the fall. Plasma volume returns toward normal with spontaneous reduction of wound oedema and reconstitution of the extracellular and plasma spaces beginning after 24–36 hours.[32]

The red cell mass is not greatly reduced, even in extensive and deep injuries. Measurements have consistently shown that immediate haemolysis of circulating red blood cells (RBC) or loss by the extravascular extravasation of red blood cells into the wound does not account for more than about 10% of the RBC mass. For this reason, the administration of RBCs to treat burn shock has been abandoned by most practitioners. Also, increasing the already elevated blood viscosity by transfusion would be expected further to impair microvascular flow.

Renal function

As noted already, a scanty, concentrated urine which contains minimal amounts of sodium (<30 mEq/l) is characteristic. Experience has shown that the consistent maintenance of urine flow rates at 0.5 ml/kg per hour in adults, although not directly reflecting the glomerular filtration rate, is in fact a reliable indicator that renal blood flow is being maintained at a level sufficient to prevent ischaemic renal injury. Oliguric renal failure, a complication which accounted directly or indirectly for the majority of early post-burn deaths in the pre-modern era is rare, if these urine flow rates are maintained. There is consensus that the urine flow rate is the best and most reliable single indicator of the adequacy of fluid resuscitation. In children of <30 kg who have a higher surface area-body weight ratio, larger urine flow rates (about 1.0 ml/kg/hour) are necessary.

At these urine flow rates, arterial blood pressure is generally in the normal range and mental status remains acceptable. Occasionally, however, the arterial blood pressure as monitored by the Riva–Rocci cuff and Doppler probe may be low. After technical measurement problems have been excluded, a trial bolus infusion of fluid (500–1000 ml in 30 minutes in adults) may be instituted and its effects on the blood pressure noted.

Summary

Burn injury alters microvascular permeability, leading to the accumulation of a plasma-like oedema fluid in the region of the burn. Effective fluid resuscitation is necessary to maintain adequate perfusion to both injured and uninjured tissues. The goal of the therapy is an appropriate physiological response. The most sensitive clinical indicator is the urine output and the rate of fluid administration must be adjusted to maintain an adequate urinary flow rate. Excessive fluid administration leads to excessive oedema accumulation and a decrease in oxygen supply to the tissues. Specific physiological effects have been discussed.

References

1 Sneve H. The treatment of burns and skin grafting. *J Am Med Assn* 1905; **65**:1.
2 Blalock A. Experimental shock VIII. The importance of the local loss of fluid in the production of the low blood pressure after burn. *Arch Surg* 1931; **22**:610.
3 Rosenthal SM, Tabor H. Electrolyte changes and chemotherapy in experimental burn and traumatic shock and hemorrhage. *Arch Surg* 1945; **51**:244.
4 Cope O *et al.* Nature of shift of plasma protein to extravascular space following thermal trauma. *Ann Surg* 1948; **128**:1041.
5 Cope O, Moore FD. Study of capillary permeability in experimental burns and burn shock using radioactive dyes in blood and lymph. *J Clin Invest* 1944; **23**:241.
6 Evans EI, Purnell OJ, Robinett PW *et al.* Fluid and electrolyte requirements in severe burns. *Ann Surg* 1952; **135**:804.
7 Reiss E, Stirman JA, Artz CP *et al.* Fluid and electrolyte balance in burns. *J Am Med Assn* 1953; **152**:1309.

8 Evans EI, Bigger IA. Rationale of whole blood therapy in severe burns; clinical study. *Ann Surg* 1945; **22**:693.

9 Moore FD. The body-weight burn budget: basic fluid therapy for the early burn. *Med Clin North Am* 1970; **50**:1249.

10 Artz CP: The Brooke formula. In: *Contemporary Burn Management*. Polk HC Jr, Stone HH (eds), pp 43–51. Little, Brown and Co., Boston, Mass.1971.

11 Scheulen JJ, Munster AM. The Parkland formula in patients with burns and inhalation injury. *J Trauma* 1982; **22**:869.

12 Baxter CR, Shires T. Physiological response to crystalloid resuscitation of severe burns. *Ann NY Acad Sci* 1968; **150**:874.

13 Schwartz S. Consensus summary on fluid resuscitation. *J Trauma* 1979; **19**:876.

14 Goodwin CW, Dorethy J, Lam V, Pruitt BA. Randomized trial of efficacy of crystalloid and colloid resuscitation on hemodynamic response and lung water following thermal injury. *Ann Surg* 1983; **197**:520.

15 Goodwin CW, Long JW, Mason AD, Pruitt BA. Paradoxical effect of hyperoncotic albumin in acute burned children. *J Trauma* 1981; **21**:63.

16 Sokawa M, Monafo W, Dietz F, Flynn D. The relationship between experimental fluid therapy and wound edema in scald wounds. *Ann Surg* 1981; **193**:237.

17 Cotran RS. The delayed and prolonged vascular leakage in inflammation. II. An electron microscope study of the vascular response after thermal injury. *Am J Path* 1965; **46**:589.

18 Brouhard BH, Carvajal HF, Linares HA. Burn edema and protein leakage in the rat. I. Relationship of time of injury. *Microvasc Res* 1978; **15**:221.

19 Harms BA, Bodai BI, Kramer GC *et al.* Microvascular fluid and protein flux in pulmonary and systemic circulations after thermal injury. *Microvasc Res* 1982; **23**:77.

20 Yoshika T, Monafo WW, Ayvazian VH *et al.* Cimetidine inhibits burn edema formation. *Am J Surg* 1978; **136**:681.

21 Pitt RM, Parker JC, Jurkovich GJ *et al.* Analysis of altered capillary pressure and permeability after thermal injury. *J Surg Res* 1987; **42**:693.

22 Arturson G. Microvascular permeability to macromolecules in thermal injury. *Acta Physiol Scand* 1979; **463**(suppl):111.

23 Monafo WW. Bari WA, Deitz F *et al.* Increase of sodium in murine skeletal muscle fibers after thermal trauma. *Surg Forum* 1971; **22**:51.

24 Moyer CA, Margraf HW, Monafo WW. Burn shock and extravascular sodium deficiency-treatment with Ringer's solution with lactate. *Arch Surg* 1965; **90**:799.

25 Leape LL. Initial changes in burns: tissue changes in burned and unburned skin of rhesus monkeys. *J Trauma* 1970; **15**:969.

26 Day C, Leape LL. Tissue sodium concentration after thermal burns. *J Trauma* 1973; **12**:1063.

27 Demling RH, Kramer G, Harmes B. Role of thermal injury-induced hypoproteinemia on fluid flux and protein permeability in burned and nonburned tissue. *Surgery* 1984; **95**:136–144.

28 Mangalore PP, Hunt TK. Effect of varying oxygen tensions on healing of open wounds. *Surg Gyn Obst* 1972; **135**:756.

29 Baxter CR, Moncrief JA, Prager MD *et al.* A circulating myocardial depressant factor in burn shock. *Res Burns* 1971; **1**:499.

30 Adams HR, Baxter CR, Izenberg SD. Decreased contractility and compliance of the left ventricle as complications of thermal trauma. *Am Heart J* 1984; **108**:1477.

31 Horton JW, Baxter CR, White DJ. Differences in cardiac responses to resuscitation from burn shock. *Surg Gyn Obst* 1989; **168**:201.

32 Pruitt BA, Mason AD. Hemodynamic studies of burned patients during resuscitation, p 83. *Research in Burns: Transactions of the Third International Congress on Research in Burns*, held in Prague, September 20–25, 1970. Bern, Switzerland, Hans Huber, 1971.

33 Monafo WW. The treatment of burn shock by the intravenous and oral administration of hypertonic lactated saline solution. *J Trauma* 1970; **10**:575.

34 Monafo WW, Chuntrasakul C, Ayvazian VH. Hypertonic sodium solutions in the treatment of burn shock. *Am J Surg* 1973; **126**:778.

35 Monafo WW, Halverson JD, Schechtman K. The role of concentrated sodium solutions in the resuscitation of patients with severe burns. *Surgery* 1984; **95**:129.

36 Virgilio RW, Rice CL, Smith DE *et al.* Crystalloid versus colloid resuscitation: is one better? *Surgery* 1979; **85**:129.

37 Caldwell FT, Bowser BH. Critical evaluation of hypertonic and hypotonic solutions to resuscitate severely burned children: A prospective study. *Ann Surg* 1979; **189**:546.

38 Graves TA, Cioffi WG, McManus WF *et al.* Fluid resuscitation of infants and children with massive thermal injury. *J Trauma* 1988; **28**:1656.

39 Merrell SW, Saffle JR, Warden GD *et al.* Fluid resuscitation in thermally injured children. *Am J Surg* 1986; **152**:664.

40 Better OS, Stein JH. Current concepts: Early management of shock and prophylaxis of acute renal failure in traumatic rhabdomyolysis. *N Eng J Med* 1990; **322**:825–828.

2

Assessment of thermal burns

D.H. AHRENHOLZ, J.B. WILLIAMS, II,
L.D. SOLEM

Introduction

Most physicians treat major burns on only an occasional basis. Thus assessment of a patient with a major thermal injury, which may be complicated by an inhalation injury or associated trauma, is often an intimidating task. Many medical personnel are overwhelmed by the initial sight and smell of a severely burned patient. However, the principles of assessment are detailed in a course for Acute Burn Life Support endorsed by the American Burn Association.[1] This course is recommended without qualification to all persons involved in the acute care of thermal injuries. The course reinforces the principle that injuries must be assessed in their order of priority. The ABCs (Airway, Breathing, Circulation) must be evaluated before the burn wounds in these thermally injured patients.

Assessment priorities

Airway

For every patient who is injured by thermal, chemical, electrical or other trauma, evaluation of the airway has first priority. Patients who have complete airway obstruction will not survive. Rapidly inspect the oropharynx for vomitus or other obstruction. The airway can be maintained by an oral obturator (Guedel type airway), or by endotracheal intubation when the presence of cervical spine injury has been excluded.

Breathing

Quickly observe the chest and auscultate the quality of breath sounds bilaterally. Chest movement with total absence of breath sounds indicates an upper airway obstruction. Unilateral absence usually indicates a tension pneumothorax or large haemothorax. Thoracostomy tube insertion can await a chest X-ray in patients who are not cyanotic or in obvious respiratory distress.

Patients with obvious evidence of an inhalation injury, respiratory distress, or circumferential neck burns, require early endotracheal intubation. Orotracheal intubation is preferred except in the presence of associated neck trauma. Facial and basal skull fractures are a relative contra-indication to nasal intubation; a cricothyroidotomy is quick, safe, and preferable to emergency tracheostomy.

Circulation

Briefly check the presence and adequacy of pulses, (radial, femoral or carotid) and obtain a blood pressure reading. Hypotension in a burn patient is almost invariably caused by hypovolaemia, either due to fluid loss into the burned tissues or secondary to a haemorrhage from associated injuries. Silent myocardial infarctions, although an uncommon complication, may also cause hypotension.

Primary assessment

All clothing is removed from the patient and the skin completely examined in a warm room. The extent of the second and third degree burns will be used to calculate the fluid requirements. Each area of the body is also quickly assessed for the possibility of associated blunt or penetrating trauma. This information is carefully documented in the medical record.

Secondary assessment

Once the physician is assured the patient has an adequate airway and blood pressure without major associated injuries, a more careful history and physical examination is obtained. Major trauma patients exhibit rapid clinical changes in the first hours and days after injury. Careful reassessment of these changes is required to treat new problems and discover injuries not apparent during the primary evaluation.

The clinical history

The medical history provides the clues to which injuries are anticipated after major trauma. The physician should complete the patient interview, as assistants place intravenous cannulae, a urinary catheter and obtain preliminary X-rays. Many major burn patients become ventilator dependent or even comatose within hours of their injury, so the entire history must be rapidly obtained from the patient. Family members and accident witnesses are also major sources of information.

Pertinent history

The history must be thorough but concise. Determine the time of the accident and the type of burning materials. Some fuels such as gasoline produce especially severe burns.[3] Vapours from burning plastics cause a chemical pulmonary injury, especially if the fire occurred in an enclosed space.[4] The risk of blunt or penetrating injury is increased if there was an explosion, if the patient jumped or fell from a burning building or was burned in a motor vehicle accident.

Immunizations

All thermal injury patients require tetanus immunization.[5] Tetanus toxoid is not repeated if the patient has been fully immunized and has had a booster within the previous 5 years. Tetanus hyperimmune globulin is given in combination with tetanus toxoid if the immunization status is uncertain.

Concurrent illnesses

List all pertinent medical conditions. A number of factors markedly increase the mortality of thermal injury, including diabetes mellitus, atherosclerosis, chronic renal failure, cirrhosis, collagen vascular disease, steroid use, malignancy, leucopaenia secondary to chemotherapeutic agents, and immunodeficiency states.[6] The risk of surgical procedures is increased in patients with ischaemic heart disease and cerebrovascular disease.

Medications

List the patient's current medications. Drugs such as steroids and cardiac medications indicate other disease states or impairment of immune function. Suspect self-inflicted injuries in patients taking psychotropic agents.[7] Suicide precautions may prevent further injury after hospitalization.

Tobacco, ethanol and drugs

A history of tobacco use increases the risk of pulmonary complications. A surprising percentage of patients sustain thermal burns as a result of ethanol or drug abuse.[8,9] Acute substance withdrawal may complicate fluid resuscitation.

Social history

List the names, addresses and telephone numbers of all close family members. They may give a history of depression or bizarre behaviour in patients who have self-inflicted thermal burns, or they may remember critical portions of the medical history. If the patient requires ventilator support, these family members will be required to make decisions regarding the care of the patient.

In severely burned adult patients, discreetly enquire if the patient has a will. If the patient spends a few minutes with a lawyer, the family may be saved endless probate difficulties should the patient ultimately succumb. Some patients with overwhelming burns may choose not to receive aggressive resuscitation.[10]

Abuse

Abuse is the cause of many thermal burns in children.[11] A careful social history may reveal abuse in other family-members or previously unexplained injuries in the victim.[12] Risk is increased for male children, less than 3 years of age, who are left with a baby sitter or boyfriend, although women also may abuse their children. A delay in seeking medical attention for the child more than 30 minutes after injury should also raise the question of abuse.[13] Specific patterns of injury have been identified. Circular burns from cigarettes, and scald burns with sharply defined margins, especially in a stocking or glove distribution, must be suspect. Perineal burns in children who are not yet toilet trained should always be reported as possible abuse.[11]

Living conditions

Burn injuries are common in the poor and the homeless. Occasionally patients lose all their possessions as the result of a house fire. The loss of pets, friends, or family members in the accident can be psychologically devastating to patients. All these factors complicate in-patient management and planning for discharge. It is difficult to plan for daily baths or wound care at home if the patient is now homeless.

Physical examination of the burn patient

Three levels of burn severity are used to describe thermal burns. The skin is reddened but does not blister after first degree or superficial burns. This type of burn is very painful to the touch, but will heal within three to six days with subsequent peeling, exactly like sunburn. These burns have few physiological effects and are ignored when calculating the size of a burn wound requiring fluid resuscitation.

Second degree or partial thickness burns blister, leaving a base which varies from red and moist to pale and relatively dry. Superficial second degree burns heal in one to three weeks without permanent scars. Deep dermal burns heal in three to six weeks but result in severe hypertrophic scars after the wounds have healed.

Third degree or full thickness burns are totally anaesthetic and involve destruction of the entire dermis. These burns are dry, leathery, and white or brown in colour. Thrombosed vessels may be visible beneath the injured skin. Third degree burns greater than three or four centimetres heal very slowly and are best treated with early excision and skin grafting.

Burn size

The dimensions of small burns are easily measured, but many burns are very large or involve multiple sites. Burn size is usually expressed as the percentage of the total body surface area (TBSA) affected. Published charts are used to diagram such burns and calculate the percentage body surface area injured.[14] Calculated fluid requirements and expected mortality are derived from this measurement.

Resuscitation

All patients with major thermal burns require fluid resuscitation. The fluid requirement is calculated from the patient's weight in kilograms and the size of second and third degree burns expressed as a percentage of the total body surface area. First degree burns are excluded. For rapid initial estimation of the burn surface area, the Rule of 9's is adequate. In an adult patient, 9% of the body is represented by each of the following: one entire upper extremity, the entire head, or either the anterior or posterior surface of each lower extremity. The anterior trunk, and the posterior trunk each represent 18%. In children these percentages change, since the head and trunk represent a larger proportion of the total body surface area. For small areas, the patient's own palm excluding the fingers represents approximately 1% of the body surface area. Accurate estimates are made with a commercial burn surface area chart (see Fig. 2.1) which must be available in every emergency department.

Fluid resuscitation is initiated via large bore intravenous cannulae which initially can be placed through burned skin. Subsequently, preference is given to unburned sites. If access is difficult, percutaneous subclavian or internal jugular vein cannulation has a lower rate of septic complications than a traditional saphenous vein cutdown.

Major versus minor burns

Small burns are treated with oral analgesia and topical antimicrobials. In selected cases burns as large as 10% TBSA in adults or 5% TBSA in children can be managed in the outpatient clinic. Even patients with small burns may require hospitalization for pain control, to educate family members in burn wound care or to protect the patient if abuse is suspected.

Minor burns involve less than 10% TBSA without involvement of the face, hands, perineum or genitalia, in patients between age 10 and 50 (Table 2.1). Regional hospitals with an interest in such care can usually manage such patients as outpatients.

A major burn is defined as any burn involving greater than 20% TBSA second and third degree burns in an adult (10% TBSA in a patient under age 10 or over age 50). Similarly, burns in critical areas including the hands, face, feet and perineum are optimally managed at a regional burn centre. Major inhalation injury, associated trauma, and chemical or electrical injuries are also indications for transfer.

Pulmonary injury

Inhalation of toxic chemicals from burning plastics is the most common cause of severe inhalation injury. Heat exchange is so efficient in the

Burn estimate and diagram
Age vs area

Area	Birth-1 yr	1 – 4 yrs	5 – 9 yrs	10 – 14 yrs	15 yrs	Adult	2°	3°	Total donor areas
Head	19	17	13	11	9	7			
Neck	2	2	2	2	2	2			
Anterior trunk	13	13	13	13	13	13			
Posterior trunk	13	13	13	13	13	13			
Right buttock	2.5	2.5	2.5	2.5	2.5	2.5			
Left buttock	2.5	2.5	2.5	2.5	2.5	2.5			
Genitalia	1	1	1	1	1	1			
Right upper arm	4	4	4	4	4	4			
Left upper arm	4	4	4	4	4	4			
Right lower arm	3	3	3	3	3	3			
Left lower arm	3	3	3	3	3	3			
Right hand	2.5	2.5	2.5	2.5	2.5	2.5			
Left hand	2.5	2.5	2.5	2.5	2.5	2.5			
Right thigh	5.5	6.5	8	8.5	9	9.5			
Left thigh	5.5	6.5	8	8.5	9	9.5			
Right leg	5	5	5.5	6	6.5	7			
Left leg	5	5	5.5	6	6.5	7			
Right foot	3.5	3.5	3.5	3.5	3.5	3.5			
Left foot									
						Total			

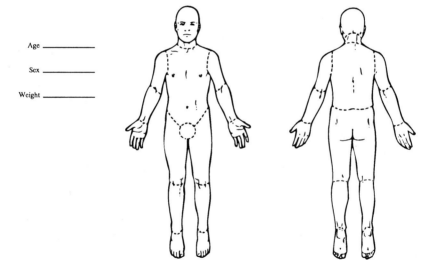

Age _____

Sex _____

Weight _____

Fig. 2.1. The Lund–Browder chart is used to calculate the size of thermal burns.[14] (By permission of *Surg Gynecol Obstet.*)

Table 2.1. *Major versus minor burn injuries*

	Age	Burn size
Minor burns		
	<10 or >50	<10%
	10–50	<20%
Major burns		
	<10 or >50	>10%
	10–50	>20%
Factors mandating admission:		
Burns of the face, hands, feet, perineum or genitalia		
Inhalation injury		
Associated major trauma		
Major concurrent medical illness		
Electrical or chemical injury		

upper airway that heat injury does not occur to the lower respiratory tract except with steam burns[15] or ignition of inhaled hydrocarbons. A brassy voice, sooty sputum, marked wheezing on chest examination, or immediate radiographic changes are more reliable signs of pulmonary injury than singed nasal hair or a blackened tongue.[16]

Diagnostic changes may not occur on chest X-ray for several hours. Most patients can be managed clinically, although some burn centres perform routine bronchoscopy to assess upper airway damage.[16]

A carbon monoxide level must be obtained in all patients with suspected inhalation injury, in addition to the routine blood gas determinations. Normal carbon monoxide levels in smokers may be as high as 6%; levels greater than 40% are associated with major central nervous system dysfunction.[17] Initially, all patients with suspected pulmonary injury must receive high-flow humidified oxygen until the carbon monoxide level is determined. The half-life of carbon monoxide in a patient breathing 100% oxygen is approximately 45 minutes. Thus if a patient arrives in the emergency room receiving oxygen therapy, it is still possible to estimate the peak carbon monoxide level.[18] Great controversy remains regarding the use of hyperbaric oxygen in the treatment of carbon monoxide poisoning.[19]

Patients with a confirmed inhalation injury must be immediately intubated and may require mechanical ventilatory support. Steroids are contra-indicated and prophylactic antibiotics are of questionable value. Inhalation injury approximately doubles the predicted mortality of a thermal burn.[20]

Monitoring

Patients with major thermal burns require large bore intravenous cannulae for fluid resuscitation and a urinary catheter. Fluid infusion is adjusted to maintain a urine output of 0.5 ml to 0.7 ml of urine per kilogram per hour in adults, or 1 ml per kilogram per hour in children who weigh less than 30 kg. A nasogastric tube relieves the gastric distension characteristic of major thermal burns. An arterial catheter is used to monitor blood pressure in patients with massive extremity oedema and for blood gas determinations in inhalation injury patients. A cutaneous pulse oximeter will continuously determine oxygen saturation. For intubated patients, an end-tidal carbon dioxide monitor is especially valuable when the patient is being weaned from ventilatory support. In a patient with normal cardiac function, a Swan–Ganz catheter is rarely necessary and has a high risk of catheter-related sepsis.[21]

Escharotomies

Circumferential third degree burns of the trunk, neck or extremities produce a band-like constriction during fluid resuscitation with impaired chest movement, upper airway obstruction, and distal ischaemia, respectively. Therefore, all patients who have circumferential third degree burns require escharotomies. Without anaesthesia the eschar is incised through the dermis to visible fat (Fig. 2.2). Incisions over the chest produce an immediate improvement in ventilation for patients with severe chest burns. Bleeding is controlled with chromic sutures or topical haemostatic agents. Pain, massive bleeding, and permanent scarring will result if the incisions are made through any area except a full thickness burn.

When thermal burns extend to muscle, swelling within the fascial sheath can produce distal ischaemia. Elevated compartment pressure measurements are an indication for emergency fasciotomies under general anaesthesia.

Associated injuries – the secondary assessment

Level of consciousness

Even the most severely burned patients are awake and alert immediately after the injury. A depressed level of consciousness is diagnostic of other problems such as acute carbon monoxide poisoning, hypoxic brain injury,

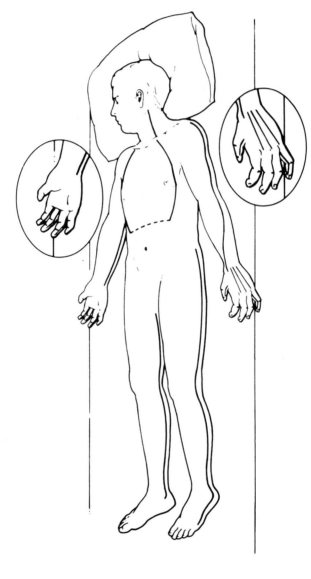

Fig. 2.2. Correct placement of escharotomy sites. Escharotomies must not be placed through unburned skin, even if the swelling is marked. Adapted with permission from McDougal, Slade, Pruitt.[22]

closed head trauma, or intoxication with alcohol or drugs. All patients with an altered sensorium must be tested for the presence of ethanol and other drugs. A gradual improvement in mental status in such patients may be followed by symptoms of acute withdrawal.

Eyes

After facial burns, carefully examine the eyes for evidence of corneal abrasion or, after an explosion, for foreign bodies and penetrating injuries. The eyes frequently swell and completely close during the first 24 hours of fluid resuscitation, precluding an adequate examination for many days.

Ears

Perforations of the tympanic membrane are common when an explosion has occurred. Even without rupture, permanent traumatic hearing loss is possible. Severe burns of the external ear predispose to the development of chondritis.[22]

Nose and mouth

Facial injuries, including nasal fractures, loose teeth, abrasions and lacerations are not uncommon if the patient has been involved in a motor vehicle accident. Subsequent facial swelling during resuscitation will make evaluation and treatment of these injuries difficult.

Chest

Fractured ribs and cardiac contusions can occur after falls and motor vehicle accidents. Careful auscultation of the chest may reveal a pneumothorax which can be confirmed with a chest radiograph.

Abdomen

Abdominal injuries are usually the result of motor vehicle and aircraft accidents, although are occasionally seen after falls from heights. Even patients who were wearing seat belts can sustain injuries, especially small bowel rupture. The abdominal examination is entirely unreliable in the immediate post-burn period. Therefore, a diagnostic peritoneal lavage, which can be carried out safely even through burned skin, must be routinely performed in patients with a possible abdominal injury.[23]

Bones

Fractures can result from a fall, a jump, an electrical injury or an automobile accident. A careful physical examination may reveal bruising, bony deformity or instability. Radiographs of the spine are also obtained to rule out compression fractures.

Re-assessment

Major thermal burn patients undergo rapid physiological changes in the first 24 hours. These include massive accumulation of oedema fluid and swelling of both burned and unburned tissue. The patient must be continuously assessed for adequacy of tissue perfusion and renal function. Secondary airway compromise must be treated early and aggressively with intubation and ventilatory support. Escharotomies and more rarely fasciotomies are required if peripheral perfusion is inadequate, but tissue swelling alone is not an indicator for such incisions. Any patient who exhibits cardiovascular instability or unexplained anaemia in the face of appropriate fluid resuscitation must be re-evaluated for the presence of undiagnosed injuries.

Electrical injuries

Electrical conduction injuries present some unique diagnostic challenges. When current flows beneath the skin, massive tissue damage may occur in the absence of cutaneous findings. This may lead to inadequate fluid resuscitation, renal failure, compartment syndromes and unnecessary tissue loss.

Conduction injuries

Patients exposed to electrical current frequently sustain thermal burns, as well as conduction injuries. The heat of the electrical arc ignites their clothing causing a secondary thermal injury. Such burns can obscure the characteristic entrance and exit or contact sites associated with electrical conduction injuries. Table 2.2 is a list of morbid signs of major electrical conduction injury. These are indications for urgent fasciotomies combined with operative debridement.

Table 2.2. *Indicators of electrical conduction injury*

Loss of consciousness or confusion (suggestive)
Cratering of entrance or exit sites
Loss of pulses or perfusion
Loss of muscle function
Mummification of digit or extremity
Flexor surface arc injuries
Myoglobinuria
Markedly elevated serum CK levels

Fluid resuscitation

In the electrically injured patient fluid requirements are determined by thermal surface burns plus any tissue injured by the electrical current. Burn surface calculations are never adequate to estimate the fluid required for resuscitation of electrical conduction injuries. Resuscitation fluid is given to obtain a urine volume of at least 100 ml per hour in adults and 1 ml per kilogram per hour in children with suspected conduction injuries.

Myoglobinuria

Myoglobinuria is diagnostic of severe muscle injury. The presence of dark coloured urine and a positive qualitative test is an indication for immediate treatment (the quantitative urine test for myoglobin often takes days or weeks to obtain). Initially, a bolus of resuscitation fluid is given followed by intravenous sodium bicarbonate to alkalinize the urine. Mannitol is administered as the urine volume begins to increase. Each hour a tube of urine is retained so that progressive clearing of the myoglobin can be observed. Persistent myoglobinuria is an indication for urgent fasciotomy, debridement or even amputation.

Associated injuries

Many major electrical conduction injuries occur while the patient is working around overhead wires. The injury often causes a loss of consciousness and a fall. The patient may be unable to give any history of the accident. Fractures of both the spine and long bones are common either from a fall or from violent muscular contractions caused by the electrical current.

Injuring voltage

In well-grounded individuals, lethal cardiac arrhythmias can occur with even 110 volt current. But major tissue injury is typically associated with high voltage currents, greater than 1000 volts.[24] Therefore, every effort must be made to determine the injuring voltage. If the signs of conduction injury are equivocal, the serum creatine kinase (CK) level may be diagnostic. Peak CK levels less than 400 I.U. are associated with minimal injury, whereas peak CK levels greater than 2500 I.U. have a very high incidence of major muscle damage.[25]

Cardiac arrhythmias

Alternating current easily causes ventricular fibrillation, at currents as low as 100 milliamperes. If a patient receives cardiopulmonary resuscitation (CPR) immediately after the onset of the arrhythmia, the survival rate is as high as 80%.[26] No other group of patients responds as well to CPR. Unwitnessed accidents with arrhythmias usually result in fatal anoxic brain injury.

After arrival at the hospital, major cardiac arrhythmias are exceedingly uncommon. Nevertheless, the patients are admitted for cardiac monitoring if an arrhythmia is documented or suspected, if there are changes on the electrocardiogram, or if the patient has sustained loss of consciousness. If the serum CK levels are normal and no arrhythmias are observed, the patient can be discharged within 24 hours.[27]

Myocardial infarction is rare after electrical injury. Elevation of the CK–MB level is not diagnostic of myocardial injury, since skeletal muscle releases large quantities of CK–MB after electrical conduction injuries.[28] Infarction is diagnosed by clinical and electrocardiographic criteria only.

Chemical burns

Chemical burns are increasingly common in industrial and agricultural environments. Immediate treatment reduces the morbidity of such injuries.[29]

General principles

A variety of chemical agents can cause injury to the human skin. The severity of the injury is determined by the chemical composition, the concentration, and the duration of contact. The most effective immediate treatment for the majority of chemical injuries is massive irrigation with water or saline. Any available water source should be used for the initial irrigation. Specific neutralizing agents for acidic and alkaline agents are usually not available and in most cases are contra-indicated because intense heat is generated by such reactions.

Special problems

Eyes

If the eye is injured with a chemical agent, copious saline lavage is performed for at least 60 minutes. A specially adapted contact lens, which can be attached to intravenous tubing, is highly effective. Topical anaesthesia is usually used before inserting this lens. Opthalmology consultation is mandatory.

Inhalation injury

A variety of chemical agents cause severe pulmonary injury. The severity ranges from the acute chemical burn of anhydrous ammonia to the sub-acute problem of silo fillers lung. Specific neutralizing agents are not available. Management involves intubation and ventilatory support. Again, steroids are contra-indicated and prophylactic antibiotics are controversial.

Summary

Thus the early management and stabilization of thermal electrical and chemical burns requires a complete initial assessment and documentation of the injuries, followed by an ongoing secondary assessment to exclude associated injuries which may be initially undetected. Specific problem management will ultimately involve a co-operative effort among a host of consulting medical personnel.

References

1 Advanced Burn Life Support Course Endorsed by The American Burn Association. Nebraska Burn Institute, 4600 Valley Road, Lincoln, Nebraska 68510.
2 Phillips TF, Goldstein AS. Airway management. In: *Trauma*, Mattox KL, Moore EE, and Feliciano DV (eds) p 132; Appleton and Lange, Norwalk, Connecticut, 1988.

3 Williams JB II, Ahrenholz DH, Solem LD *et al.* Gasoline burns: The preventable cause of thermal injury. *J Burn Care & Rehabil* 1990; **11**:446–50.

4 Prien T, Traber DL. Toxic smoke compounds and inhalation injury – a review. *Burns* 1988; **14**:451–60.

5 Furste W, Aguirre A, Lutter KS. Tetanus. In: *Surgical Infectious Disease.* (2nd edn). Howard RJ and Simons RL (eds) pp 837–847, Appleton and Lange, Norwalk, Connecticut, 1988.

6 Zawacki BE, Azen SP, Imbus SH *et al.* Multifactorial probit analysis of mortality in burned patients. *Ann Surg* 1979; **189**:1–5.

7 Klasen HJ, Van Der Temdel GL, Hekert J *et al.* Attempted suicide by means of burns. *Burns* 1989; **15**:88–92.

8 Berkelman RL, Herndon JL, Callaway JL *et al.* Fatal injuries and alcohol. *Am J Prev Med* 1985; **1**:21–8.

9 Parks JG, Noguchi TT, Klatt EC. The epidemiology of fatal burn injuries. *J Forens Sci* 1989; **34**:399–406.

10 Imbus SH, Zawacki BE. Autonomy for burned patients when survival is unprecedented. *N Eng J Med* 1977; **297**:308–11.

11 Purdue GF, Hunt JL, Prescott PR. Child abuse by burning – an index of suspicion. *J Trauma* 1988; **28**:221–4.

12 Hight DW, Bakalar HR, Lloyd JR. Inflicted burns in children: Recognition and treatment. *J Am Med Assn* 1979; **242**:517–20.

13 Hobbs CJ. When are burns not accidental? *Arch Dis Childh* 1986; **61**:357–61.

14 Lund CC, Browder NC. Estimation of areas of burns. *Surg Gyn Obst* 1944; **79**:352–8.

15 Moritz AR, Henriques FC, McLean R. Effects of inhaled heat on air passages and lung; experimental investigation. *Am J Pathol* 1945; **21**:311–31.

16 Hunt JL, Agee RN, Pruitt BA. Fiberoptic bronchoscopy in acute inhalation injury. *J Trauma* 1975; **15**:641–9.

17 Winter PM, Miller JN. Carbon monoxide poisoning. *J Am Med Assn* 1976; **236**:1502–4.

18 Clark CJ, Campbell D, Reid WH. Blood carboxyhaemoglobin and cyanide levels in fire survivors. *Lancet* 1981; **i**:1332–5.

19 Ellenhorn MJ, Barceloux DG (eds): Medical toxicology. pp 820–835. In: *Diagnosis and Treatment of Human Poisoning.* Elsevier, New York, NY; 1988.

20 Shirani KZ, Pruitt BA, Mason AD. The influence of inhalation injury and pneumonia on burn mortality. *Ann Surg* 1987; **205**:82–7.

21 Ehrie M, Morgan AP, Moore FD *et al.* Endocarditis with the indwelling balloon-tipped pulmonary artery catheter in burn patients. *J Trauma* 1978; **18**:664–6.

22 McDougal WS, Slade CL, Pruitt BA. In: *Manual of Burns*, McDougal WS, Slade CL, Pruitt BA (eds) pp 136–137, Springer-Verlag, New York, NY, 1978.

23 Ward H, Ahrenholz DH, Crandell H *et al.* Primary closure of wounds in burned tissue: Experimental and clinical study. *J Trauma* 1985; **25**:125–7.

24 Solem LD, Fischer RP, Strate RG. The natural history of electrical injury. *J Trauma* 1977; **17**:487–92.

25 Ahrenholz DH, Schubert W, Solem LD. Creatine kinase as a prognostic indicator in electrical injury. *Surgery* 1988; **104**:741–7.

26 Moran KT, Thupari JN, Munster AM. Electric- and lightning-induced cardiac arrest reversed by prompt cardiopulmonary resuscitation (letter). *J Am Med Assn* 1986; **255**:2157.

27 Purdue GF, Hunt JL. Electrocardiographic monitoring after electrical injury: Necessity or luxury. *J Trauma* 1986; **26**:166–7.

28 McBride JW, Labrosse KR, McCoy HG *et al.* Is serum creatine kinase – MB in electrically injured patients predictive of myocardial injury? *J Am Med Assn* 1986; **255**:764–8.

29 Curreri PW, Asch MJ, Pruitt BA. The treatment of chemical burns: specialized diagnostic, therapeutic, and prognostic considerations. *J Trauma* 1970; **10**:634–42.

Transportation

D.L. EDBROOKE, R.E. JOHN, R.J. MURRAY

Introduction

The transportation of the thermally injured patient may be divided into primary transport, i.e. that between the site of injury and the receiving hospital, and secondary transport, i.e. between the receiving hospital and the specialist burn unit. The necessary level of expertise and the equipment required are different in the two situations. It must never be assumed that burns will be the only injury present.

Primary transportation

The initial call

The initial call will reveal the location, the number of injuries, the cause and type of injuries, the approximate time of the incident, the type of environment the incident occurred in, and the identity of the person reporting the incident. This information will aid in decisions regarding the personnel, vehicles, equipment and protective clothing that must be sent. If indicated, other services must be informed at this stage.

Arrival on scene

Vehicles must be parked where they are out of danger and not blocking essential access or exits. The priority is to communicate with the emergency services on scene, and establish who is in charge. Introduce yourself, listen to their report of the situation, and together decide a plan of action. Safety of the team is paramount. Seek expert advice on the safety of buildings, natural hazards, explosion risks, or the spread of fire and smoke. At all times, maintain communication between ambulance control and the receiving hospital.

Assessment and treatment at site

Assess first who is injured, then the severity of injury. The number of casualties must be ascertained and a formal triage performed. Delegate tasks to others as appropriate. Each patient then must be assessed in more detail once triage has been undertaken. The initial assessment has been dealt with in the chapter on Assessment. It is vitally important to maintain body temperature, but contaminated clothing must be removed. If clothing has been removed, foil blankets or other warm coverings must be used to conserve body heat. Burned areas can be covered in 'clingfilm' which will decrease heat loss, decrease painful contacts, and aid analgesia. It will also be possible to visualize the wound in the receiving hospital without removing the dressing. Wet dressings are not advised as these will vastly increase heat loss, and this will increase mortality and morbidity in traumatized patients.

Early pain relief is important. Intravenous opioids are the treatment of choice, but must only be administered by those appropriately trained. Patients that are hypoxic or hypovolaemic may show confusion or agitation. Such patients may be very sensitive to the effects of opioids, and their use may complicate the situation. Each patient must have a case record attached which will include presumptive diagnoses, basic observations and treatments given with the time and doses noted.

Stabilization of the patient before transport may be advisable in certain cases, such as treatment of life-threatening arrhythmias after an electrical injury. However, trauma victims with internal injuries will benefit from rapid, skilful transfer to the receiving hospital where specialist treatment can be instituted.

Transportation

The patients must be monitored throughout the journey. Treatment including additional analgesia must be continued en route as necessary. Transfer itself can exacerbate the existing deleterious physiological changes. The parameters that should be monitored continually during transfer are listed in Table 3.1.

It is vital to communicate with the driver so that the speed of the vehicle can be adjusted to the needs of the patient. It is still a commonly held

Table 3.1. *Parameters to be monitored during primary transport*

Respiratory rate and pattern
Heart rate and rhythm
Capillary refill time
Blood pressure
Level of consciousness
Blood and fluid loss
Oxygen saturation

belief that the faster the drive the better the outcome: this is not necessarily the case.

Handover

There is often poor co-ordination between the primary care worker and the receiving hospital. Verbal communication is neither reliable nor accurate, and must be backed up by carefully written notes. Additional history from witnesses, relatives, fire service, police or ambulance crews is important.

On arrival at the Accident and Emergency Unit, the patient must be placed in a warm environment and fully re-examined with clothing removed. The primary care worker must introduce him/herself to the admitting team and remain during this examination, drawing attention to injuries already identified. Only after this is completed can they leave.

Secondary transportation

Secondary transportation occurs between the receiving hospital and a specialist centre, in this case a Burns Unit. The condition of the patient has been stabilized as far as possible, and definitive treatment is required which cannot be undertaken at the unit initiating primary treatment. The decision to transfer a patient must be made by a senior doctor, following consultation with the specialist unit.

Stabilization prior to transfer

Before secondary transportation, it is vital that the patient is fully assessed and resuscitated. The value of this in preventing cardiovascular and respiratory disasters has been established in many publications.[1–3] A full survey of the patient must be carried out. Consider a patient with burns who has also ruptured his spleen in a fall. He may die from massive haemorrhage during transfer. The burns become a secondary consideration: he needs an urgent laparotomy, transfusion, reassessment and then transfer.

Biochemical and haematological parameters must be optimized. For example, it is dangerous to transfer patients in whom the serum potassium is acutely abnormal as this will predispose to arrhythmias. Equally, transferring a hypoxic patient increases the risk. Arterial blood gas and carboxyhaemoglobin estimation must, if possible, be performed prior to transfer.

Airway problems need managing definitively prior to transport. It is unacceptable to allow the development of airway obstruction during transfer. Any suggestion of airway involvement must alert the transfer team to the need for intubation prior to leaving. Oropharyngeal oedema associated with burns is progressive and is at a minimum during the initial period of resuscitation. The longer the delay, the more difficult intubation will become. Once intubated, formal positive pressure ventilation must be initiated. There is no place for intubated patients breathing spontaneously during transfer. This implies the presence of someone trained in the care of the unconscious, ventilated patient.

Attention must be given to the dressing of wounds, the immobilization of fractures and the continuation of appropriate analgesia and sedation. Escharotomy of circumferential burns may be necessary.

The risks of transfer must be balanced very carefully against the possible benefit. There is no place at this stage for impulsive action.

Preparation for transfer

Before transfer all relevant personnel including the receiving unit, ambulance service, airforce and police must be properly briefed regarding the timing and method of transport.

Personnel must be selected well in advance and must be familiarized with the patient. Inexperienced personnel must not be left in charge.

It is the responsibility of the personnel transporting the patient to ensure that all necessary equipment is present and in full working order. The equipment taken must be sufficient to allow the management of most eventualities. For example, during the transfer of a ventilated patient with head injuries it would be prudent to include a chest drain, as a pneumothorax could occur.

A versatile and complete pre-packed transfer kit must always be available. This kit must be routinely checked and maintained. A great deal of thought must be given to the preparation of this kit. Decisions must not be made 15 minutes prior to transportation (Appendix 3.1).

Drugs and equipment that definitely will be required during transfer must be packed separately so as not to deplete the kit unnecessarily. It is useful to have muscle relaxants, analgesics and sedatives drawn up in syringes, and to have the next bag of intravenous fluid readily available.

Check that enough oxygen is present, not only for the transfer, but making allowances for unforeseen delays.

Prepare a formal written summary of the injuries and management for presentation to the receiving team upon arrival. All relevant documentation (including investigation results and X-rays) must be carefully packaged and accompany the patient.

The transfer

If adequate attention has been given to the preparatory phase then some of the problems commonly associated with transfer may be avoided. It must be borne in mind that the environment within a transfer vehicle is less forgiving than that of a hospital facility. Routine tasks are hampered by the effects of this environment. For example, limited access, noise, motion and impaired visibility can make the measurement of blood pressure impossible. Communication difficulties, electrical interference, and temperature changes can present problems particularly during air transportation. Transportation by air must be considered, but safety, costs and work space area must be taken into account (Appendix 3.2).[4]

It must be appreciated that there is always an element of isolation from the support normally available within hospitals. This feeling is unfamiliar to most hospital doctors.

Once aboard the vehicle, ensure that staff, equipment and patient are in the best possible position. The equipment must be secured to avoid injury. Access to the patient needs thought, as does the safety of the staff.

Physiological changes occur as a direct result of transportation. As yet much work remains to be done in this field but an outline of the major problems are summarized below.

It has been well documented that patients being transferred can suffer tachycardia and hypertensive episodes.[5] This is often accompanied by cardiac arrhythmias particularly those with recent evidence of myocardial infarction.[6] These changes can be attenuated by attention to oxygenation, sedation and analgesia.

Hypotension may also occur in patients who have previously been stable, caused by fluid shifts secondary to acceleratory and deceleratory forces. An additional fluid load may be necessary before they are moved. Fluid regimes must be assessed, and delivery using a volumetric pump with battery backup will ensure that the required volumes are given in the specified times. A urinary catheter must be inserted before transfer, and fluid balance charts must be kept.

Patients transported without adequate airway control are at severe risk of hypoxia.[7] This is diminished if the airway is controlled, but there is evidence that moderate hypoxia and hypercarbia can still occur.[8,9] There is some dispute as to whether manual control of ventilation is preferable to the use of a portable ventilator. The ideal appears to be hand ventilation with a method of monitoring tidal volume at the expiratory valve.[10] Practicalities however must be considered and it would appear sensible to opt for a portable ventilator, allowing free hands to perform other tasks without interrupting ventilation.

The maintenance of body temperature is vitally important in patients suffering from burns and/or multiple trauma. The victim must be well shielded from the elements and all must be done to protect them from heat loss. 'Clingfilm' and foil blankets must be used. The vehicle must be warmed, and the amount of time between vehicle and building or in the cold accepting area minimized.

There is a wealth of literature describing the effects of hypertension and hypoxia on the intracranial pressure but little is known about the effects of transport *per se* on this. Practically, it would appear that the cardiovascular and respiratory systems must be stabilized to reduce the changes in intracranial pressure. Sedation and analgesia are important adjuncts in avoiding these changes, and the choice of any agent will be a personal preference guided by the condition of the patient.

Handover

The same principles apply as in primary transport. Again it is important that all documentation is given to the admitting team together with a verbal report. It is the responsibility of the doctor transferring the patient to ensure that the patient is formally handed over to the appropriate member of the admitting team.

Summary

It is important to plan the whole exercise carefully and in advance. Predictable problems that can occur during transportation must be avoided and adequate preparation should reduce the effects of less predictable problems. The safety of patients must be given consideration, as must the safety of the staff. Good communication is vital at all times if the best interests of the patient are to be properly served. It is likely that with the increase in financial constraints the incidence of transportation will increase. With careful attention to detail, an associated potential increase in morbidity may be avoided.

References

1 Macdonald RC, Banks JG, Ledingham I McA. Transport of the injured. *Injury* 1981; **12**:225–33.
2 Bion JF, Edlin SA, Ramsey G, McCabe S, Ledingham I McA. Validation of a prognostic score in critically ill patients undergoing transport. *Br Med J* 1985; **291**:432–4.
3 Ehrenwerth J, Sorbo S, Hackel A. Transport of critically ill adults. *Crit Care Med* 1986; **14**:534–7.
4 Baack BR, Smoot III E, Kucan JO *et al.* Helicopter Transport of the patient with acute burns. *J Burn Care & Rehabil* 1991; **12**:3, 229–33.
5 Insel J, Weissman C, Kemper M, Askanasi J, Hyman A. Cardiovascular changes during transport of critically ill and postoperative patients. *Crit Care Med* 1986; **14**: 539–42.
6 Taylor JO, Landers CF, Chulay JD, Hood WB, Abelman WH. Monitoring high-risk cardiac patients during transportation in hospital. *Lancet* 1970; **ii**:1205–8.
7 Gentleman D, Jennett B. Hazards of interhospital transfer of comatose head injured patients. *Lancet* 1981; **ii**: 853–5.
8 Indeck M, Peterson S, Smith J, Brotman S. Risk, cost and benefit of transporting ICU patients for special studies. *J Trauma* 1988; **28**:1020–5.
9 Waddell G, Scott PDR, Lees NW, Ledingham I McA. Effects of ambulance transport in critically ill patients. *Br Med J* 1975; **1**:386–9.
10 Gervais HW, Eberle B, Konietzke D, Hennes H, Dick W. Comparison of blood gases of ventilated patients during transport. *Crit Care Med* 1987; **15**:761–3.

Further reading

Medical Aid at Accidents, Roger Snook MD. Update Publications.
ABC of Resuscitation 2nd edn, edited by F.R. Evans, BMJ Publications. ISBN 0-72979-0260-1.
Anaesthesia for the Surgery of Trauma. Clinic Anaesthesia Services. Edited by A.H. Geisecke, ISBN 8036-4100-1.
Ellis A, Rylah LTA. Transfer of the thermally injured patient. *Br J Hosp Med* 1990; **44**: 206–8.

Appendix 3.1.

Equipment for out-of-hospital use

The exact constitution of 'out-of-hospital' care kits varies. Their weight and volume will be determined by the circumstances under which they will be used.

No attempt is made to describe a kit that can be used under all circumstances, as no such thing exists. Rather, suggestions regarding items which may prove useful or essential will be listed. There are differences in the contents, weight and packaging of kits intended for inter-hospital transfer and use in other circumstances. A kit intended for use during inter-hospital transfer may be totally unsuitable for field situations such as helicopter evacuation from ships.

Packaging is important. Solid cases provide the best protection for inter-hospital transfer kits; however, soft waist-carried pouches are more suitable for field use.

Tightly packed boxes reduce dimensions for carriage, but impair access to a greater extent than a loosely packed compartmented structure. Typed waterproofed lists of the contents of each container will facilitate use and aid restocking. Two or three medium-sized cases are better than one large unmanageable container.

First aid equipment

Sterile gloves
Wound dressings
Burns dressings (plus fluid if appropriate)
Bandages
Adhesive tape
Safety pins
Mosquito forceps
Scissors
Povidine–iodine spray
Antiseptic solutions

Airway management

Self-inflating bag
Masks, of various sizes
Oxygen enrichment system, and tubing
Sterile gloves

Portable suction
Suction catheters
Airways (oro- and naso-pharyngeal) of various sizes
Endotracheal tubes (cut and uncut) of various sizes: contained in a roll for
  rapid deployment
20 ml cuff-inflating syringe
Artery forceps
Endotracheal tube ties (pre-cut)
1″ Adhesive tape
Right-angled, double-swivel connector
Catheter mount
Disconnecting wedge
Intubating stillettes
Gum elastic bougie
Magill forceps
KY jelly
Laryngoscope handles
Laryngoscope blades (Macintosh sizes 3 and 4, paediatric blade, e.g.
  Robertshaw)
Spare batteries and bulbs
Cricothyrotomy and tracheostomy equipment
Oesophageal obturator
Laryngeal masks
Nasogastric tubes
Throat pack
Oxygen masks and tubing
Nebulizer set
Portable ventilator

Intravenous fluid therapy

Cannulae of various sizes
CVP Cannulae
Skin-prep swabs
Tourniquet
Sterile gloves
Cut-down set
Adhesive tape
Tincture of benzadine
Suture material (adhesive tape does not work in the rain)
Elbow immobilizer
Gauze swabs
Fluid administration sets
Bungs
Fluid: Ringer's lactate, gelatins, hetastarch, dextrose
Pressure infusor
Syringes and needles
Cross match bottles and request forms
Hooks for bags of fluid
Fluid warming pouch
Battery operated infusion pumps

Chest drainage

Chest drains of various sizes
Heimlich valves
Collecting bags
Suture material
Adhesive tape
Scalpel
Large clip
Sterile gloves
Sterile drape

Drugs

Oxygen (cylinders, reducing valves, piping, cylinder keys, etc)
Entonox kit
Ketamine
Thiopentone
Etomidate
Suxamethonium (powdered form for long-term storage, or obtain fresh supply
  from hospital fridge)
Vecuronium
Nalbuphine
Morphine (stored separately in locked container with drug register to comply
  with legal requirements)
Naloxone
Prilocaine
Diclofenac
Droperidol
Metoclopramide
Diazepam
50% glucose
Glucagon
Adrenaline
Atropine
Calcium
Lignocaine
Bicarbonate
Propranolol
Verapamil
Flecainide
Hydrocortisone
Dexamethasone
Frusemide
Chlorpheniramine
Ranitidine
Aminophylline
Salbutamol: inhaler, nebulizer and IV
Saline (100 ml bags store easily)
Water
Antibiotics
Ampoule file
Syringes and needles
Syringe labels

Diagnostic and monitoring

Stethoscope
Aneroid sphygmomanometer and cuffs
Blood glucose estimation sticks
Thermometer
Tendon hammer
Opthalmoscope and auroscope kit
Defibrillator/ECG with gel pads, leads, etc
Non-invasive automatic blood pressure monitor
Pulse oximeter

General

Warm clothing
Waterproofs
High visibility, reflective tabard
Gloves
Hard hat/helmet
Boots
Powerful hand torch
Head torch
Spare batteries and bulbs
Heavy-duty scissors (for removal of clothing, boots, etc)
Space blankets
Pens/pencils
Chinagraph pencils
Triage labels
Notepaper and envelopes
Casualty record sheets
Dictaphone
Camera, with flash equipment, film and batteries
Portable anaesthetic equipment (e.g. the Triservice apparatus)
Equipment for local anaesthetic blocks
Emergency surgical equipment, e.g. amputation set
Mast (Military anti-shock trousers)

Vehicle

Flashing beacon
Two-way radio
Siren
Fire extinguisher
Reflective warning triangles

The following items are usually carried by the other emergency services:

Rigid cervical collars
Spinal immobilization for extrication
Splints
Casualty insulation bag
Blankets
Stretcher
Mobile shelter
Cutting and extrication equipment

Appendix 3.2.

Air transportation

Transportation by air has the advantage of speed when the distances involved
are great. Fixed wing transportation is usually quicker than rotary wing
transportation (600–120 mph v 200–70 mph) but this advantage is often lost in
lengthy transfers to the airstrip.

Rotary wing flights are at lower altitude and consequently present few of the
problems associated with reduced atmospheric pressure. However, turbulence
and dependence on weather conditions are a problem. Fixed wing aircraft do
not present major problems if they are pressurized as the cabin pressure does
not usually exceed 8000 ft. Care must be taken in unpressurized aircraft to
avoid hypoxia. Consequently, consultation with the flight crew is essential
regarding maximum effective altitudes. The air in the cuffs of endotracheal
tubes should be replaced with saline to minimize volume changes in the cuff.

In all forms of air transportation, communication is a major problem. Noise
is a particular problem in helicopters. Another major practical problem is space
making good planning prior to travel a necessity. Electronic medical equipment
may be in close proximity to the electronic instrumentation of the aircraft or
helicopter. This may produce interference.

It is worthy of note that there is a stepwise increase in cost. Helicopter
transportation is many times more expensive than fixed wing transportation
which, in turn, is many times more expensive than ground transportation. This
factor has to be taken into account in the decision-making process.

4

Resuscitation of major burns

J.L. HUNT, W.W MONAFO, G.F. PURDUE,
L.T.A. RYLAH

Introduction

There are many ways to resuscitate a major burn injury. This chapter will cover the three most widely used methods. First, there will be a short recapitulation of the pathophysiology and the general physiological principles involved. Then the 'Parkland', the 'Hypertonic lactated saline', and finally the 'Muir and Barclay' formulae will be described. The monitoring and assessment of a successful resuscitation for each formula will be explained in a pragmatic fashion. It is hoped that this will enable the reader to perform a successful resuscitation, no matter which path is chosen.

Pathophysiology

Both local and systemic alterations to physiology occur after a thermal injury. The greater the injury, the more marked the alterations. Immediately, post-burn haemodynamic stability is reflected by a normal blood pressure, a slight tachycardia, and an increased respiratory rate. Within several hours the cardiac output will fall, the severity of the fall being dependent on the size of the burn. There will be a compensatory increase in peripheral resistance to maintain a normal blood pressure. The initial depression of cardiac output will occur before any significant hypovolaemia.[1] Isotonic fluid is sequestered into the burn wound and also into non-burned tissue. Hypovolaemic shock would soon occur if the intravascular volume was not repleted. Cardiac output slowly returns to near normal levels within 24 hours in all but the largest burns.

Fewer than 3% of all acute burns die from hypovolaemic shock and acute renal failure. These 'resuscitation failures' generally occur in burns exceeding 90% body surface area. Patients with pre-existing cardiac or renal disease may have an uneventful resuscitation when adequate intravenous fluids are administered promptly.

An understanding of the changes occurring in the microvasculature helps to explain the large volumes of fluid needed to resuscitate the burned patient. An immediate capillary leak occurs in the burn wound. In large burns a generalized leak occurs even in the unburned areas. A rapid and massive shift of fluid from the intravascular to extravascular interstitial space results in progressive oedema formation. The capillary leak is greatest during the first eight hours post-burn. The capillary integrity is slowly regained and is back to normal by 18 to 24 hours post-burn. It can thus be seen that the two important goals of early burn care are the prompt initiation of resuscitation and an adequate volume replacement regime. A more detailed description is to be found in Chapter 1.

General principles

If possible, intravenous access is established by percutaneous cannulation, preferably through unburned skin. However, if suitable sites are not available, there is no contra-indication to intravenous access through burned skin. Peripheral sites are always attempted before choosing a central location. All patients requiring intravenous resuscitation must have two large bore cannulae (minimum 16 gauge) inserted. The length of the catheter will affect the rate of infusion, and thus long multi-lumen, or long central venous catheters are not recommended for this purpose.[2] If immediate intravenous access is needed, and no other site available, a central vein, either femoral or jugular (internal or external) must be used.[3] It is wise to reserve the subclavian route for hyperalimentation, or monitoring with a flow-directed pulmonary artery catheter. The potential risk of a pneumothorax in a hypovolaemic patient must be weighed against the potential advantages of such techniques.[4] All intravenous access lines, both central and peripheral, must be changed and rotated to a different location every three days to minimize the risk of suppurative thrombophlebitis or septicaemia.

Baseline parameters must be obtained on admission. These will be plasma sodium, potassium, chloride, bicarbonate, urea, creatinine and glucose. The haemoglobin, haematocrit, white cell count and a baseline for clotting function must be determined. Arterial blood gases and carboxyhaemoglobin are obtained in all intubated patients, those with or suspected of having an inhalation injury, or chronic lung disease.

Formal resuscitation is carried out in all adults with burns over 15–20%. Superficial or first degree burns are excluded. The 'Rule of nines' (see Chapter 2) can be used to calculate the percentage total body surface area (% TBSA) burned in people over the age of 15. The patient's actual weight is calculated by subtracting the urine output from the amount of fluid given, then subtracting this number from the admission weight. (1 litre = 1 kilogram).

$$Wt(kg) = \text{Admission weight} - (\text{Fluid given} - \text{urine output})$$

Monitoring

Blood pressure is monitored hourly by a non-invasive technique or continuously by an indwelling arterial cannula. Errors can occur when measuring the blood pressure in a burned arm. The cuff must be large enough to encircle 80% of the upper arm. If the arm is burned, the circumference will increase during resuscitation due to oedema forma-tion and the cuff may become too small. Blood pressure will be dampened if the cuff is placed on either an oedematous arm or over thick eschar. An arterial line is inserted in most burns over 40% and in all intubated patients. Peripheral sites for arterial cannulation are always selected first, and unlike venous lines, are not routinely changed unless they mal-function.

The most reliable clinical parameter for evaluating the response of the patient to resuscitation is urine output. This applies to all formulae. In adults, 0.5 ml/kg/h of urine is the goal. A urine output in excess of this, in the absence of glycosuria or diuretics, indicates a need to reduce the rate of infusion. An adequately resuscitated patient at the end of 24 hours should have a clear sensorium, normal blood pressure, a pulse rate less than 120 per minute, and a minimal base deficit (2–3 mmol/litre).

Frequently, excessive urine outputs are encountered. Common reasons include over estimation of either the burn size or depth, the weight, an incorrect intravenous rate, or glycosuria. It is not unusual to encounter a mild 'stress' pseudo-diabetes. The serum glucose will be 9–10 mmol/litre. This is occasionally seen for several hours during the early phase of resuscitation. Glycosuria will be absent or mild, but is usually transient and will require no treatment.

Serial haematocrit (Hct) determinations are of little value as a guide to adequacy of resuscitation. Haemoconcentration will occur because of the capillary leak but no loss of red cell volume. In burns larger than 50%

TBSA, the Hct will continue to rise during the first 24 hours post-burn in spite of large fluid infusions, and it may exceed 55 or 60%.

During the first 24 hours of resuscitation, the cardinal clinical sign of hypovolaemia is a urine output of less than 0.5 ml/kg/h. Confusion, anxiety, restlessness, obtundation (in the absence of hypoxaemia, sedation or an intubated patient) a base deficit greater than 5 mmol/l, a serum bicarbonate less than 16 mmol/l, or a core/peripheral temperature difference of over 5 °C, are other clinical signs of hypovolaemia.

The Parkland formula (Hunt & Purdue)

The Parkland formula[5] calls for 4 millilitres of Ringer's lactate per kilogram per % TBSA burn to be infused over 24 hours.

$$4 \times \text{weight in kilograms} \times \% \text{ TBSA (ml)}$$

This generally is the only electrolyte solution used during the first 18–24 hours of resuscitation. The electrolyte content of Ringer's lactate in mmol is sodium 130; potassium 4; calcium 3; chloride 109; bicarbonate 28. Although slightly hypotonic, the solution closely approximates the composition of the extracellular fluid. It is a balanced salt solution with a ratio of lactate (a bicarbonate precursor) to chloride similar to that of extracellular fluid (27 : 103). In addition each litre contains approximately 80–100 ml of free water. The latter is ideal for replacement of the electrolyte free portion of maintenance fluid. Although the solution has a pH of 5.1, this has little effect on the blood pH. Even when large volumes are infused, the lactate is rapidly converted to bicarbonate.

One half the calculated amount or 2 ml/kg/ % TBSA burn is given over the first 8 hours after the burn. The remaining half is then administered equally over the next 16 hours. This formula is used only to estimate requirements. Hourly urine measurements are the best way to monitor the patient's response to resuscitation. In adults urine output is maintained at 0.5 ml/kg/h. Since the fluid determined by the formula is only to be used as an initial guide, the patient must be continually assessed. The infusion rate will have to be adjusted frequently during resuscitation. All intravenous fluids must be pre-warmed.

Following a normal resuscitation, the functional extracellular fluid volume is restored to nearly normal, or to 20% of the body weight in kilograms. However, plasma volume remains low and is not corrected, regardless of the amount of crystalloid administered. Colloid will not remain in the intravascular space during the first 8 hours post-burn. Over the next 16 hours the capillary integrity improves and most colloid will remain in the intravascular space. Generally, patients with burns under 30% do not develop a clinically significant plasma volume deficit.

Fresh frozen plasma (FFP), 0.5 ml/kg/ % TBSA burn, is administered between 22 and 24 hours post-burn. The typical clinical response after colloid administration is an abrupt increase in urine volume and a decrease in pulse rate. In the majority of resuscitations early administration of colloid is unnecessary. Fresh frozen plasma is used because it furnishes the needed oncotic effect, contains the important clotting factors V and VIII, and fibronectin, an important opsonin which is deficient in the early post-burn phase.

If FFP is unavailable, plasmanate or purified plasma protein fraction (5% human USP; human albumin solution 4.5% BP) is also effective. These are heat-treated products with no hepatitis infection risks. Human albumin (25% USP; 20% BP) may also be used for volume expansion, by mixing 100 ml of the 20% or 25% albumin with crystalloid, in a ratio of 1:3 or 1:4 and administering 0.5 ml/kg/ % TBSA burn.

If excessive urinary output is encountered, the infusion rate is decreased for the next hour by an amount equal to the excess urine volume. For example, if the expected urine volume was 50 ml per hour, and the actual was 150 ml, the infusion rate is decreased by 100 ml per hour. Administering fluids at a rate in excess of that needed to maintain normal hourly urine results in the majority of the fluid passing into the extravascular space and exaggerating oedema formation.

Table 4.1. *Conditions associated with excessive fluid requirements*

Delayed initiation of resuscitation
Inadequate early volume replacement
Inhalation injury
Deep burns
Electrical burns
Topical enzymatic debriding agents
Malnutrition and liver disease

Approximately 15% of the patients admitted to Parkland require more fluid and 12% of patients less fluid than the amount calculated by the formula. Certain clinical conditions are associated with fluid requirements in excess of that calculated by the formula (Table 4.1). The presence of an inhalation injury deserves special comment. Fluid requirements will be in excess of that calculated by the Parkland formula. The greater the magnitude of pulmonary injury, the greater the fluid requirements.[6] The patient must never be intentionally resuscitated on the 'dry' side.[7]

When urine output is less than anticipated for 2 consecutive hours, the infusion rate is doubled and the patient re-evaluated in 1 hour. An intravenous bolus of fluid is never given as sudden increases in intravascular pressure will drive more fluid into the extravascular space. Colloid is administered in any patient that shows clinical hypovolaemia and exceeds the crystalloid requirement by one and a half times that calculated at the 12 to 18 hour post-burn stage. If urine output still remains less than desired, resuscitation requirements must be re-evaluated. The patency of the urinary catheter must be checked, otherwise, the burn size must be recalculated, and the patients weight must be reassessed.

While clinical estimation of intravascular volume at the end of the first 24 hours is inexact, the above mentioned guidelines are adequate in the majority of cases. If these causes have been excluded, then more exact monitoring of cardiac function is necessary. A pulmonary artery catheter must be inserted at this stage.

Less than 1% of all acute admissions require invasive monitoring during this period. Indications include clinical evidence or suspicion of hypovolaemia after administration of one and a half to two times the calculated volume at 12 to 18 hours post-burn, evidence of myocardial failure, or any patient, especially the elderly, with old or recent myocardial infarction. A pulmonary artery catheter (Swan–Ganz), not a central venous line, must be utilized, as more useful haemodynamic parameters are available.

The pulmonary capillary wedge pressure (PCWP) is the most useful parameter to assess volume status. Fluid is administered to maintain a normal PCWP (12–15 mmHg). If urine output continues to remain inadequate and the cardiac output remains low, inotropic cardiac support must be considered as a matter of urgency. The peripheral resistance will be elevated, but vasodilator therapy is contra-indicated because of the rapidly changing volume status of the patient. It is inappropriate to administer additional fluid because of a low PCWP when the urine output is adequate. Each case must be evaluated on its own merits and no dogmatic resuscitation guidelines regarding monitoring are appropriate.

Potassium, other than that in Ringer's lactate, is not given in the first 24 hours post-burn. Although serum potassium usually remains normal, it is monitored closely because an intracellular deficit will develop during this period. Amounts often exceeding 50 to 80 mmol per litre are excreted in the urine. Potassium replacement therapy will usually be needed during the second 24-hour period post-burn.

24 to 48 hours post-burn

At the end of the first 24 hours, crystalloid is stopped and only 5% dextrose solution in water (D5W) is administered. The serum sodium is maintained in the range 130–133 mmol per litre. Sufficient sodium has been administered, and it becomes more important to replace evaporative water losses occurring through the burn wound. Dextrose solution (5%) is initially infused at a volume of 1 ml/kg/ % TBSA/day. Serum sodium must be measured at least every 24 hours.

In burns greater than 60% TBSA, clinical signs of hypovolaemia may still be evident after 48 hours. This may indicate a persistent plasma volume deficit and the need to administer additional colloid. Since the exact amount is unknown, one half the amount given at the end of the first 24 hours is given. The patient's vital signs and urine output are constantly re-evaluated. A spot urine sodium is a helpful qualitative diagnostic tool to evaluate intravascular volume. A value greater than 20 mmol per litre, if no diuretic has been given, is suggestive of an adequate intravascular volume. Less than 5 mmol per litre indicates renal sodium conservation and volume depletion.

A spontaneous post-resuscitation urinary diuresis begins about the fourth or fifth post-burn day as the extravascular burn oedema is mobilized and reabsorbed into the intravascular space. Urine volumes in excess of 150 ml per hour are common, gradually returning to normal over the next few days. The patient's weight should be close to the pre-burn weight by day 7 to 10 post-burn. During this diuresis the intravascular volume will become depleted if the metabolic fluid requirements are not sufficient.

The post-burn diuresis may be delayed, blunted, or absent altogether if surgery is performed during the first five days.[8] This is especially common after full thickness burn wound excision. The removal of a large amount of oedematous burn eschar and subcutaneous tissue eliminates fluid that would normally be mobilized and excreted.

Hypertonic lactated saline (HLS) solutions (Monafo)

Although resuscitation with lactated Ringer's solution is indeed highly effective in preventing early death, there has been concern about possible

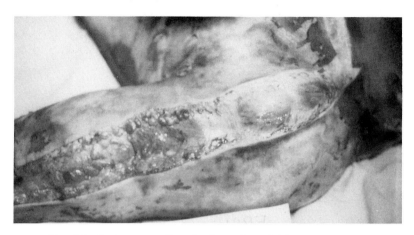

Fig. 4.1. Escharotomy lines in circumferential burns.

complications from the large volumes of fluid commonly required. The burn wounds typically become turgid and tense. This increased tissue pressure may impair the already compromised circulation in tissues immediately adjacent to the burns. Thus, partial thickness burns may be converted to full thickness injuries that will require skin grafting. Morbidity and mortality rates are directly related to the extent of full thickness injury. Furthermore, mobilization of the accumulated oedema may lead to cardiopulmonary insufficiency in the post-resuscitative phase. In addition, severe oedema underlying unyielding full-thickness circumferential burns of the limbs may result in muscle compartment syndrome, and circumferential burns of the torso may restrict ventilation as oedema accumulates. Both scenarios are common in practice, such that limb or truncal escharotomies are frequently necessary in patients with circumferential burns resuscitated with lactated Ringer's solution (Fig. 4.1). As long as these oedema related complications are recognized promptly, they can be treated effectively by escharotomy or fasciotomy. If performance of these procedures is delayed, irreversible underlying tissue injury may occur with loss of limb or digit. However, these procedures themselves may complicate wound management by opening sub-escharotic planes and predisposing to invasive burn wound sepsis.

Because of these concerns, clinicians have long had an interest in minimizing the total fluid volume administered to burn patients. Based on early experimental data suggesting that hypertonic saline solutions could be used effectively to treat burn shock, Monafo began to use such solutions over 20 years ago.[9,10] In a recent series, both isotonic and

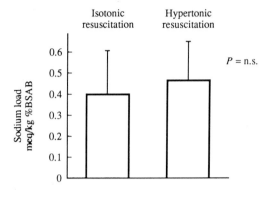

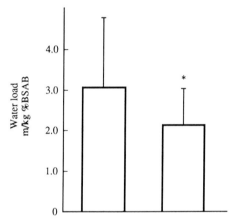

Fig. 4.2. Comparison of normotonic and hypertonic fluid loads during resuscitation.

hypertonic saline solutions were administered to patients acutely follow-ing burn injury in volumes sufficient to maintain urine flow and other parameters as outlined above.[11] In the first 24 hours post-burn the total sodium load was similar with all solutions but the total fluid volume required was reduced by as much as 40% when hypertonic solutions were used (Fig. 4.2).

The solution is formulated by adding 100 mmol of racemic sodium lactate to 1 litre of normal saline. The resultant mixture contains 254 mmol of sodium, 154 mmol of chloride, and 100 mmol of lactate. The goals of resuscitation are exactly the same as those already discussed.

Fluid is administered at a rate sufficient to maintain the urinary output at the desired level, starting at 0.3 ml/kg/ % TBSA burn to be given in the first hour, and then adjusted accordingly (i.e. 70 kg person with a 50% TBSA burn needs $0.3 \times 70 \times 50 = 1050$ ml). Moderate degrees of hypernatraemia and hyperosmolality are common, especially in patients with extensive injuries and large fluid requirements. However, this is usually well tolerated. Plasma concentrations of sodium and potassium and osmolality must be determined every 4–6 hours in severe injuries. If the sodium concentration exceeds 155 mmol/l and/or the plasma osmolality exceeds the 340–350 mosm/l, the hypertonic infusion must be reduced or discontinued, and a less concentrated sodium solution administered as required to maintain the specified urinary output.

In patients with overt shock at the time of presentation, it is generally preferable to infuse lactated Ringer's rapidly to achieve the desired blood pressure and/or urine output. Then administration of the HLS may be initiated. Infusion rates greater than 1 litre/hour should be avoided. The hypertonic solution must be discontinued when the phase of extravascular fluid flux has abated, usually after 24–36 hours.

When HLS is used for fluid resuscitation in burn shock, these additional clinical guidelines should be observed:

1. Major burn injuries often coexist with acute alcohol intoxication or following the ingestion or transcutaneous absorption of other compounds which may elevate plasma osmolality. Administration of concentrated sodium salt solutions in this setting would be unwise. Thus, in addition to the history, a baseline determination of serum osmolality must be performed routinely prior to, or immediately after the institution of HLS therapy. If the serum osmolality is high, HLS must be withheld.
2. The mental status of the patient must be monitored closely. In our experience, however, alterations in mental status attributable to elevated osmolality and dehydration of the CNS have not occurred provided the serum sodium concentration and osmolality remain within the limits described.
3. HLS may be administered either into a peripheral vein or into the central venous circulation.
4. Periodic blood samples for electrolyte and osmolality determinations must not be drawn proximal to (downstream from) the intravenous line through which HLS is being administered. This could affect the measured values and mislead the clinician.

5. Patients with extensive burns (75% TBSA or greater) will require more fluid administration than patients with lesser injuries and therefore will be at greater risk for developing hyperosmolality and hypernatraemia. Thus, when modest elevations in these parameters occur in these patients (especially sodium >150 mmol/l and/or osmolality >320 mosm/l), it is often prudent to alternate HLS with lactated Ringer's on a 1-to-1 or 1-to-2 basis.

6. When the phase of extravascular fluid flux has abated, it is imperative that sodium-free water (5% dextrose solution) be administered following the discontinuation of the HLS infusion. This is necessary to replace the increased evaporative water loss from the wound and to prevent the development or exaggeration of hypernatraemia. Oral fluids must be given as soon as is feasible. One of the apparent advantages of HLS therapy is that gastrointestinal function is preserved or returns promptly following the phase of extravascular fluid flux. The continued administration of saline solutions in the post-resuscitative phase, which is usually indicated by a falling haematocrit, is usually unnecessary and will promote additional wound and soft tissue oedema. Older patients especially will avidly retain whatever sodium and water loads have been given. The mobilization of this excess oedema will be prolonged and may place patients at increased risk for cardiopulmonary dysfunction.

7. If the urine output should fall off after the first 48 hours post-burn, a gentle diuresis may be induced with frusemide BP (furosemide USP) 5–10 mg intravenous, or a similar agent. A brisk response to this small dose of diuretic attests to the adequacy of the intravascular volume and to the abundance of the extracellular fluid.

The use of hypertonic saline solutions according to the above guidelines is safe. Effective resuscitation can be accomplished with a decreased volume of fluid and with less wound oedema than are required with other fluid regimens. If fluid resuscitation has been accomplished successfully and carefully, and if no other complications such as sepsis intervene, the patient's body weight should approach pre-burn values within 5–7 days post-burn.

Muir and Barclay formula (Rylah)

The aim of the Muir and Barclay[12] formula is exactly the same as the other formulae, that is to maintain tissue perfusion especially to the kidney, heart and brain. To accomplish this, a solution of 4.5% human albumin solution is infused, and equal amounts of this fluid are given over six periods of time. These consist of three periods of 4 hours, then two periods of 6 hours, and finally one period of 12 hours. This gives a resuscitation time of 36 hours, beginning at the time of the injury. The amount of fluid given per period in millilitres is equal to half the product of the percentage body surface area burned (% TBSA) multiplied by the weight in kilograms.

$$0.5 \times \text{weight (kg)} \times \text{\% TBSA each period (ml)}$$

A urinary catheter is inserted into the patients bladder and hourly urine measurements are taken. The aim is a urine output of 0.5 ml/kg/hour. If the output is much lower than this target, the volume given in the next hour is increased by one half. A bolus of fluid will increase oedema formation in a similar fashion described in the Parkland technique. If the hourly urine is excessive, the infusion fluid is decreased by one half.

The metabolic fluid needs have not been taken into account and must be supplied. Dextrose 4%, saline 0.18% solution BP is administered at a rate of 1.5 ml per kilogram per hour. The metabolic needs for smaller adults and children can be ascertained by using the formula:

> 100 ml per kg up to 10 kg body weight and then
> 50 ml per kg from 10 kg to 20 kg and then
> 20 ml per kg thereafter, given equally over a
>   24-hour period.

The original formula stated that the haematocrit must be measured at the end of each period. However, the haematocrit will always tend towards being high, which will result in a larger volume than necessary being infused. Similarly, chasing a low central venous pressure or pulmonary wedge pressure will result in unnecessary high volumes being infused. The singular most important measurement is the hourly urine output. It must be remembered that the formula is a starting point and only a guide. The patient must be constantly re-assessed and a dynamic fluid replacement regime instigated.

Younger patients will maintain central perfusion in the face of gross volume deficits by vasoconstriction. This will become evident by a large difference between the core and peripheral temperatures. If resuscitation is progressing well but peripheral temperatures are low, it would be wise to increase the colloid to aid peripheral perfusion. Core temperature will rise to approximately 38.5 °C and peripheral to within 3 or 4 °C of that, if adequate volume replacement is given.

The blood pressure if measured will be normal, or low normal if vasodilation has occurred. There will be evident a tachycardia of 110–120 beats per minute. Greater than this signifies a volume deficit or another pathology, e.g. pain, infection, respiratory distress, etc which must be diagnosed and acted upon. There may be a tachypnoea and it is advisable to commence oxygen therapy at an early time. Pulse oximetry will guide the clinician to the relevant inspired oxygen concentration, as would blood gas analysis if oximetry is not possible or unavailable. The monitoring of the more difficult case has been explained earlier and does not differ in any aspect.

There will be less fluid infused during resuscitation when compared to a crystalloid technique. There will therefore be less oedema, and fewer airway problems. However, that oedema which does form takes longer to subside as protein has to be mobilized from the extracellular space. Respiratory problems are no more frequent, but tend to last longer when colloid is administered. It is obvious that any crystalloid technique will cost less to administer than colloid, and with a single fluid regime, it may be safer when used by inexperienced operators than a mixed regime of crystalloid and colloid.

Historical perspective

In 1942 Harkins[13] recommended 100 ml of plasma/ % TBSA burn. Then in 1952 Evans *et al*[14] used a formula of 1 ml of plasma plus 1 ml of 0.9% saline/ % TBSA/kg body weight. Sorenson (1971)[15] used Dextran 70 in a 6% solution made up in 0.9% saline at a rate of 120 ml/ % TBSA burn in 24 hours less that volume given by mouth. Pruitt and Welch in 1977 described the Brooke Army Hospital formula[16] as 1.5 ml Ringer's lactate and 0.5 ml plasma/% TBSA burn/kg plus 2 litres of 5% dextrose in water by mouth. Most of these formulae have fallen by the wayside, but may still be used by some centres.

Future developments

It is clear from the diversity of formulae and fluids that not one of the methods is superior to another. In the past 10 years, other fluids for volume expansion and resuscitation have come on the market. The dextrans have almost been abandoned due to allergic reactions. It has been found that up to 70% of the population have an immunoglobulin which causes this reaction but not all of these 70% will react unfavourably.

The gelatins, both urea linked and succinylated, have a molecular weight which makes their plasma volume replacement too short lived. They will cause an osmotic diuresis which may interfere with the vital signs. They do not interfere with haemostasis but the urea-linked gelatins have calcium in the solution, which may interfere with blood transfusions. There has been some concern for their use in burns as they decrease fibronectin levels and therefore may interfere with wound healing and by decreasing opsonin levels interfere with the immune response.

The most promising compounds seem to be the starches.[18] These are produced by the reaction of ethylene oxide on amylopectin to produce hydroxyethyl starch (HES). These compounds are classified by their molecular weights and degree of substitution. At present the most usable compound is 6% Hetastarch (MW 450 000; substitution 0.7). This compound produced as Hespan (DuPont) closely mimics 4.5 or 5% albumin, and has been substituted for such. Other forms of starches are available, i.e. Elohes 6% (200 000:0.62)[17] which has a much shorter half-life, or Pentastarch (250 000:0.45) which is very similar in physical properties. A refined form of pentastarch called pentafraction has an average molecular weight number of 120 000 and a degree of substitution of 0.45. This has been shown to decrease the fluid load in an animal model and may be shown to have a worthwhile clinical application in the future.

Summary

The three most commonly used formula for resuscitation have been described in a pragmatic way which will help the resident to follow a successful resuscitation through to the end. The monitoring and clinical aspects of resuscitation have been explained and an insight into future developments given.

References

1 Baxter, CR. Problems and complications of burn shock resuscitation. *Surg Clin Am* 1989; **58**:1313–22.
2 Selwyn A, Russell WJ. Flow through cannulae. *Anaesth Intens Care* 1977; **5**:157–60.
3 Purdue GF, Hunt JL. Vascular access through the femoral vessels: Indications and Complications. *J Burn Care & Rehabil* 1986; **7**:498–500.

4 Feliciano DV. Major Complications of percutaneous subclavian vein catheters. *Am J Surg* 1979; **138**:869.

5 Baxter CR. Early resuscitation of patients with burns. In: *Advances in Surgery*, 4. Welch CE (ed). Year Book Medical Publishers, Chicago. 1970.

6 Navar PD, Saffle JR, Warden GD. Effect of inhalation injury on fluid resuscitation requirements after thermal injury. *Am J Surg* 1985; **150**:716–20.

7 Herndon DN, Traber DL, Traber LD. The effect of resuscitation on inhalation injury. *Surgery* 1986; **100**:248–50.

8 Frame JD, Taweepoke P, Moiemen N, Rylah LTA. Immediate fascial flap reconstruction of joints and use of Biobrane in the burned limb. *Burns* 1990; **16(5)**:381–4.

9 Monafo WW. The treatment of burns shock by the intravenous and oral administration of hypertoniclactated saline solution. *J Trauma* 1970; **10**:575.

10 Monafo WW, Chuntrasakul C, Ayvazian VH. Hypertonic sodium solutions in the treatment of burn shock. *Am J Surg* 1973; **126**:778.

11 Monafo WW, Halverson JD, Schechtman K. The role of concentrated sodium solutions in the resuscitation of patients with severe burns. *Surgery* 1984; **95**:129.

12 Muir IKF, Barclay TL: *Burns and Their Treatment*. Lloyd Luke Ltd, London 1974.

13 Harkins HN: *The Treatment of Burns*. Chas. C Thomas. Springfield, Illinois. 1942.

14 Evans EI, *et al.* Fluid and electrolyte requirement in severe burns. *Ann Surg* 1952; **135**:804.

15 Sorensen B. Fluid therapy with Dextran. In: *Contemporary Burn Management*. Polk CH and Stone HH (eds). Little, Brown & Co., Boston 1971.

16 Pruitt BA, Welch GW. *The Burn Patient in the Intensive Care*. Kenney MJ, Bendixen HH, Powers SR (eds). W.B. Saunders Co. Philadelphia, PA, 1977.

17 Bennett ED, Vincent JL (eds). Fluid replacement with ELOHES. A new hydroxy-ethyl starch solution. *Supplement to Clinical Intensive Care*, Vol 2, No. 1. Castle House Publications Ltd, 1991

18 Webb AR: The physical properties of plasma substitutes. *Clin Intens Care* 1990; **1**: 58–61

5

Inhalation injury

W.R. CLARK

Introduction

Injuries which result from smoke inhalation occur in victims with and without thermal injuries to the skin. These injuries may involve the upper airway (larynx, trachea, and bronchi) or lower airway (pulmonary parenchyma) alone or together.[1] The clinical consequences of injuries at these different anatomical sites are not necessarily concurrent or of equal severity. Heat *per se* is thought to be responsible for only a small portion of these injuries; the primary mechanisms of injury depend on tissue exposure to the chemical species resulting from incomplete combustion. The chemistry of smoke is extraordinarily complex;[2] even though the toxicology of smoke is probably not as complex as its chemistry, toxicological studies have not led to the development of treatment strategies useful to the clinician. In spite of many circumstantial speculations, the sequence of pathophysiological events which leads to the clinical state of most smoke inhalation victims is unknown.[3,4]

The literature on smoke inhalation is confusing because of the frequent lack of adequate definitions, diagnostic imprecision, a wide range of injury severity, and the failure to differentiate between respiratory insufficiency due to smoke inhalation from that which is a consequence of one or more of the many pulmonary complications of thermal injury alone.[3] The causes of these include fluid overload, massive transfusion, prolonged anaesthesia, sepsis, aspiration, pneumonia, etc.

This chapter will attempt to clarify some of the issues mentioned above and provide some practical guidelines for the assessment and management of patients suspected or known to have a smoke inhalation injury. Smoke refers to the airborne products of incomplete thermal degradation of material.[2] This chapter will confine itself to the treatment of victims of a single exposure to smoke from unwanted and uncontrolled fires. It will not address the problems caused by exposure to cigarette smoke, smog, chemical fumes, or the repetitive exposures which occur in firefighters. 'Smoke inhalation injury' constitutes an injury to the proximal airway or pulmonary parenchyma severe enough to result in detectable clinical consequences.[3,5,6] The range in toxicity of smoke and the vulnerability of individuals is so wide that 'smoke exposure' is often not associated with significant symptoms.

Epidemiology

The thermal decomposition of material may be accompanied by flames (combustion) or be without flame (pyrolysis); the potential for injury exists in both conditions.[2] Furthermore, smoke moves easily in response to winds and drafts so that injury can occur at sites remote from the fire. The hypoxia resulting from the carbon monoxide and cyanide compounds in smoke interferes with correct perceptions and reduces physical capacity which are the reasons for the inappropriate responses and feeble escape efforts often seen. Smoke reduces visibility and is a powerful conjunctival irritant thus interfering with both escape and rescue. Many smoke victims do not survive long enough to enter the health care system.[7] Carbon monoxide alone is responsible for over half of these fatalities; burns account for only 10–20% of them. The role played by acute alcoholism, coronary artery disease, pre-existing illness, cyanide, heavy metals and other toxins in these deaths is significant though not clearly defined.

Clinical presentation

The condition in which smoke inhalation victims present to the emergency department is extremely variable.[3,8,9] Some arrive in cardio-respiratory arrest, respond to resuscitative efforts, but remain brain dead due to prolonged hypoxia. Others enter with partial obstruction of the upper airway with hoarseness, stridor, retraction, wheezing, bronchorrhoea, and spasms of coughing. Individuals with a latent injury often have little or no dyspnoea when first seen and are without laboratory or imaging abnormalities, but progress to a state of florid respiratory failure some 6–36 hours later. Often indistinguishable from these when first seen are the patients who present with transient symptoms of conjunctival and upper airway irritation and become asymptomatic rapidly. The many variations on these scenarios merge with them to form a spectrum of injury severity which is wide.[8,9] Patients anywhere on this spectrum may present with or without a skin burn; when present the burn is invariably a flame injury and thus often significant. Among burn and smoke victims admitted to hospital, approximately 15% have both burns and some degree of smoke exposure or injury; about 5% have a problem only as a result of smoke inhalation without a burn. The mortality rate for the former group ranges from 29–50%, that for the latter is about 8%.[6,8] This suggests that the smoke-injured lung is more vulnerable than the healthy lung to the inflammatory and septic stress imposed upon it as a result of the burn wound.[8,10] The oedema which is a consequence of adequate resuscitation in burn victims contributes to the obstructive component of inhalation injuries and interferes with the patients' ability to clear their secretions and maintain an airway.[11]

Diagnosis

The diagnosis of inhalation injury is occasionally obvious, occasionally difficult; in the latter instance it will depend on inferences from indirect evidence and sequential assessments during an interval of observation. More frequently, it falls somewhere between these two extremes. A high index of suspicion, assessment of pre-hospital events, and determination of the patient's premorbid respiratory status are critical to diagnostic precision and optimal care.[8,11,12]

The diagnostic characteristics of smoke inhalation patients in the categories of history, physical examination, laboratory evaluation and chest imaging are presented in Tables 5.1–5.4. This data is based on a study of 108 patients.[8]

Burns of the face by themselves do not correlate well with the presence of an inhalation injury because they are present in many patients without smoke inhalation.[8] Carbonaceous sputum produced by almost half of patients correlates well with bronchoscopic evidence for soot in the proximal airway.[13]

Elevated levels of carboxyhaemoglobin (CoHgb) result in hypoxia responsible for the profound metabolic acidosis often present in these patients on admission.[8] However, the arterial oxygen partial pressure (PaO_2) is normal prior to the advent of alveolar collapse and reflects the oxygen content of the inspired gases. The normal PaO_2 may mitigate the tachypnoea which might otherwise be present because the carotid body is more responsive to arterial oxygen tension than arterial oxygen content.[14] Elevated levels of CoHgb serve as indirect evidence for exposure to combustion products. Normal CoHgb levels do not rule out an inhalation injury, especially if the interval between exposure to smoke and blood sampling is greater than 4–6 hours or shorter if oxygen has been administered.[8,15] There is no correlation between CoHgb levels and hospital mortality or respiratory failure.

The initial chest radiograph is often of poor technical quality because of portable technique and patient movement; it is rarely abnormal possibly because subtle changes are missed.[8,16] Abnormalities on subsequent films may reflect complications of thermal injury (i.e. aspiration, fluid overload, pneumonia) as easily as smoke inhalation. Xenon[133] ventilation scans are positive in a high proportion of these patients although their lack of specificity is a problem in patients with pre-existing chronic lung disease.[8,17] The results of this imaging technique do not correlate with injury severity, and should not control treatment, so the effort and risk involved in moving a critically ill patient to the nuclear medicine department should rarely be undertaken even when the diagnosis of inhalation injury is uncertain.

Bronchoscopic findings do not correlate well with mortality, severity of respiratory failure, or the duration of endotracheal intubation.[18,19] There is a 96% correlation between a positive bronchoscopy and the history of exposure to fire in a closed space, CoHgb greater than 10 percent and carbonaceous sputum.[13] Because of this observation and the fact that the need for intubation of the airway should be established on clinical grounds, bronchoscopy is not essential in these patients. However, the information bronchoscopy provides about the severity of laryngeal injury may be useful in weighing the relative merits of trans-laryngeal intubation versus tracheostomy in those patients who require invasive airway support.[20]

Other modalities for the diagnosis of smoke inhalation including enzymatic changes, pulmonary function changes, and cytological changes detectable following broncho-alveolar lavage have been reported.[11] For the most part, these tests require special expertise or equipment, are not instantly available, and, like many other tests, do not have a high degree of specificity in clinical practice and so are unable to prove the presence of smoke inhalation.

The gaps in our diagnostic capacity relative to inhalation injury put a premium on experience and leave the clinician with the major problem of identifying victims who present with occult injuries which are destined to become life threatening over the course of 48 hours.[21] The solution to this problem rests on a high index of suspicion, complete patient assessment and observation for as long as 48 hours.[8,11,12] Failure to anticipate major respiratory problems in these patients delays treatment which sets the stage for a prolonged illness or even a fatality. The corollary is that treatment must be vigorous and comprehensive so as to shorten the illness and forestall its progression to irreversible respiratory failure. All patients with smoke inhalation, even those who appear brain dead or hopelessly ill, must be treated aggressively during the interval of access to the health care system and initial stabilization so that as the clinical scenario unfolds, strategic decisions based on the patient's prognosis are not hampered by the uncertainties posed by incomplete resuscitation. When faced with continued diagnostic uncertainty, or failure to improve, treatment should be instituted.

From this point forward, this chapter will address the practical management of a smoke inhalation victim with a burn. A moderate degree of injury severity is assumed. The reader is asked to scale the therapeutic response up or down, depending on the requirements of the particular patient. Special considerations posed by the smoke inhalation victim without a concomitant burn will be mentioned.

Pre-hospital care

At the scene

The patient must be removed far enough from the fire site so that no further contact with smoke is possible. Any smouldering clothing must be extinguished or removed quickly while the airway is being assessed and maintained. The way this is done will vary with the needs of the patient and the capacity of the emergency medical team. Because the hypoxia consequent on lowered ambient oxygen concentration, carbon monoxide, hydrogen cyanide, breath-holding, and laryngospasm constitutes the most urgent priority of treatment, oxygen must be delivered by mask at the highest possible concentration. A global assessment keyed to the adequacy of the airway, level of consciousness, severity of burn, associated injuries, and pre-existing illness is then done to determine the priority of triage and the urgency of transport to the appropriate emergency department. The ideal emergency department needs to be staffed and equipped for the provision of comprehensive care so that definitive assessment and treatment can be started without delay. Ground transport is usually adequate if transportation time is less than 90 minutes.

During transport

Constant vigilance is required because of the threat of vomiting or cardio-respiratory arrest. Active voice control and reassurance of these patients who are frequently agitated (often inebriated) is more effective than restraints, or sedatives and narcotics, which must not be used in the un-resuscitated burn victim. Patients often cough most effectively in the sitting position which should be permitted. Oxygen delivery must be maintained.

Emergency department

In the emergency department, it is important to treat the patient continuously throughout the process of re-evaluation and diagnosis. The patient must be in a warm environment without extraneous traffic where informed surveillance is available. Warmth and moisture are added to the inspired gases at this point to help avoid bronchospasm and reduce the inspissation of bronchial secretions. The patient must be allowed to change position frequently and to sit up to facilitate coughing and expectoration. Limited suctioning of the mouth and pharynx being careful to avoid laryngeal stimulation (because of the hazard of laryngospasm) is often helpful. Patients who have survived a cardio-respiratory arrest or who have received oxygen by mask for a prolonged interval frequently have significant gastric dilation. The stomach needs to be decompressed with a nasogastric tube to eliminate this as an impediment to ventilation and reduce the chance of vomiting with aspiration.

History

The history should emphasize certain key points relative to the diagnosis of inhalation injury (Table 5.1), its severity and comprehensive patient management in the event endotracheal intubation precludes further communication. They are listed with an indication of their significance or usefulness:

1. Fire site: significant injury more frequent in closed spaces.
2. Fuel and combustion process: synthetic material and incomplete combustion often present more potential for pulmonary parenchymal injury. Smouldering combustion often linked to prolonged exposure versus explosion.
3. Duration of exposure: relates to smoke dose.

 4. Loss of consciousness: if preexisting relates to duration of exposure, if result of smoke exposure relates to severity of hypoxic episode.
 5. Method of escape: indicates degree of incapacitation.
 6. Time of exposure: allows estimate of maximum CoHgb level.[15]
 7. Treatment: has oxygen been given as in No. 6, above; or, with opiate analgesia the possible need for a narcotic antagonist.
 8. Hoarseness: indicates laryngeal involvement.
 9. Improved or worse since rescue: progression of illness.
10. Last oral intake: need for gastric emptying and calibre of tube.
11. Other pains: associated injuries, myocardial infarction.
12. Preexisting illness: degree of visceral compromise, e.g. respiratory insufficiency.
13. Medicines taken: relates to above, also steroid or thyroid dependency.
14. Drug allergies: avoid iatrogenic injury.
15. Addiction: anticipate withdrawal syndrome.
16. Possibility of assault or suicide: need for patient protection.
17. Will to live: a requirement for patient motivation.

Table 5.1. *Historical observations**

Criteria	% Present
Exposure to smoke	100
Unconscious	30
Exposure >10 minutes	19
Other death	17
Other diagnosis of smoke inhalation	15

Note: *61% of patients had two or more factors present.
Source: Adapted from *J Burn Care & Rehabil* **10**:52–62, 1989, with permission.

Physical examination

The physical examination must be focused on the respiratory system and the burn (Table 5.2) with a quick but not cursory screen for associated injuries, level of consciousness, appropriate affect and neurological impairment.

The most urgent concern in these patients relates to patency of the upper airway and adequacy of ventilation. Decisions about patient

Table 5.2. *Physical examination findings**

	% Present
Burn, face	84
Carbonaceous sputum	48
Soot, nose and mouth	44
Wheeze	31
Rhales, ronchi	23
Voice change	19
Corneal burn	24
Singed nasal vibrissa	11
Cough	9
Stridor	5
Dypsnoea	3
Intraoral burn	2

Note: *15% of patients had only one
physical finding present; 56% had three or
more findings present; 32% had four or
more findings present.
Source: Adapted from *J Burn Care &
Rehabil* **10**:52–62, 1989, with permission.

management with regard to these two issues depend entirely on clinical
assessment: history and physical examination. The diagnosis of smoke
inhalation is not the critical factor on which these decisions depend;
bronchoscopy is rarely required to make the correct decision.[20,22] Only
15% of all burn and smoke victims require intubation, and only about 5%
require this intervention on the day of injury.[20] Of all patients with an
inhalation injury or significant smoke exposure 49% require intubation
(62% for those with a burn, 12% for those without a burn).[9,20,22] About
40% of these patients require intubation to secure the airway, 5–10%
because of inadequate ventilation, the remainder because of respiratory
failure.[20] Patients requiring urgent intubation are those who:

1. are unconscious, obtunded, or suffer neuromuscular impairment;
2. are in profound shock or exhibit haemodynamic instability with
   the possibility of smoke inhalation;
3. cannot dispose of their secretions or cough effectively;
4. have significant burns or oedema of neck, face, mouth, or
   pharynx;
5. have hoarseness, stridor or are labouring to breathe.

The oedema resulting from thermal and/or chemical injury to the upper airway, face, and neck increases with resuscitation peaking at the second or third post-burn day. This oedema may compromise the airway as well as limit the patient's ability to extend his neck, open his mouth, and handle his secretions without aspiration.[20] It is critical that decisions about endotracheal intubation be made by experienced persons who can accurately anticipate the magnitude of this oedema. Airway compromise can be definitively treated with an endotracheal tube.[20] Delay in instituting this treatment creates the chance that critical airway compromise will be unrecognized[22] or that endotracheal intubation will either be technically impossible or a *tour-de-force* which carries an increased risk of further laryngeal trauma or other complications[20] associated with difficult intubation. If in doubt, intubation is the safest course of action.

Diagnostic measures

The diagnostic approach to these patients attempts to document their hypoxic stress and assess the degree of pulmonary parenchymal compromise which causes respiratory failure. Most of these tests and examinations provide indirect evidence on which inferences about inhalation injury can be based.[8,11,12,22] Many of them establish the baseline status required to monitor the patient's progress or lack of it. Few of them are critical to acute patient management, and not one of them must be allowed to compromise the quality of ongoing treatment.

Arterial blood gases must be obtained with a notation as to the oxygen concentration of the inspired gas so as to allow estimation of ventilation/ perfusion (V/Q) mismatch, shunt (Qs/Qt) or calculation of the PaO_2/FiO_2 ratio which correlates well with the more exacting Qs/Qt measurement.[23] A PaO_2/FiO_2 ratio (mmHg/decimal fraction) below 400 is abnormal, a value below 200 is an indication of serious respiratory insufficiency requiring mechanical ventilation with positive end-expiratory pressure (PEEP) to prevent further alveolar collapse and recruit atelectatic alveoli.[24] The degree of metabolic acidosis or respiratory alkalosis reflects the hypoxic stress experienced by the patient (Table 5.3). Blood is also tested for percentage of haemoglobin in the CoHgb form (abnormal > 5% in smokers[15]) and cyanide levels (abnormal > 0.20 mg/l)[25] to measure the causative agents for this hypoxia and to infer the potential for the development of severe pulmonary parenchymal failure. Pulse oximeters do not detect CoHgb and give a falsely elevated reading for oxygen saturation in its presence.[26-28] The development of pulmonary parenchymal failure is often delayed 24 to 72 hours in these patients; prior to this, the PaO_2 may be normal. The oxygen saturation calculated from this PaO_2 and haemoglobin concentrations will be normal even with high levels of CoHgb. The true status can only be demonstrated if the oxygen saturation is measured directly with a CO-oximeter.

Table 5.3. *Laboratory observations*

	% Present
CO2 < 15 mmol/l	59
CoHgb > 5% < 20%	51
(A-a) > 100 mm Hg	39
CoHgb > 20%	31

Note: CoHgb: Carboxyhaemoglobin; A-a: alvolear–arterial oxygen pressure difference.
Source: Adapted from *J Burn Care & Rehabil* 1989, **10**:52–62, with permission.

Other examinations

Pulmonary imaging examinations and bronchoscopy have been discussed earlier. In the unusual event that the initial chest X-ray shows severe parenchymal abnormalities which can be presumed to result from smoke exposure the inhalation injury is severe (Table 5.4). Most of these patients will have been intubated on clinical grounds prior to the availability of the X-ray report.

Treatment

Vascular access and resuscitation

The initial vascular access should utilize a peripheral vein and be well secured. Early efforts to place a central venous catheter are often difficult

Table 5.4. *Imaging observations*

Imaging mode	% Positive
Chest X-ray	8
Xenon–133 scan	86
Albumin scan	82

Source: Adapted from *J Burn Care & Rehabil* **10**:52–62, 1989, with permission.

because of severe hypovolaemia; hazardous, because of patient agitation increasing the risk of pneumothorax; and require putting the patient in the head down position which interferes with ventilation and often with oxygen administration. The type and volume of fluid administered must be chosen to achieve optimal resuscitation as quickly as possible. Patients with inhalation injury and a burn can be expected to require more fluid than one would expect on the basis of the burn alone;[29,30] those without a burn usually require maintenance fluid volumes only. There is no evidence that sub-optimal fluid volumes limit the degree of respiratory insufficiency which develops.[29,31] To the extent this kind of fluid regimen provides only marginal perfusion of viscera and the burn wound, it sets the stage for untreatable complications as this lengthy illness unfolds. On the other hand, excessive fluid and the bolus form of fluid administration which increases pulmonary microvascular pressure transiently must be avoided if possible.[30,32]

Bronchospasm

Wheezing may be due to oedema of the airway or mucosa, retained secretions, bronchospasm, or combinations of these factors. It can be treated with intravenous aminophylline (slow bolus 5 mg/kg followed by an infusion of 0.5 to 0.9 mg/kg/h). Blood levels of the drug need to be monitored (therapeutic range 10 to 20 μg/ml). Racemic epinephrine (adrenaline) or beta$_2$ adrenergic agonists can be administered by nebulizer. They are not always effective and must be discontinued if no benefit is detected but may be used again later in the illness if needed.

Retained secretions

Mucolytics (*N*-acetylcysteine) may be tried in an effort to break up inspissated secretions or casts of bronchial mucosa.[33] However, the mainstay in the prevention of this problem is adequate humidification of inspired gases, adequate systemic hydration, frequent position changes, vigorous chest physiotherapy, frequent endotracheal suctioning, and fibre-optic bronchoscopy when other methods fail. Suctioning and bronchoscopy in the intubated patients must be performed through a tightly fitting port in the ventilator tubing so that respiratory support and PEEP can be maintained.

Airway compromise

As noted above, endotracheal intubation is the definitive treatment for existing or anticipated airway compromise. This procedure can be extraordinarily difficult in burn victims; for this reason it is imperative that a major effort be made to optimize conditions and secure the help of the most experienced operator available so as to reduce the incidence of complications and further laryngeal trauma.[20,34] The route of intubation must depend on the preference of the intubator influenced by the location of any facial burn and the patient's clinical status. Sedation (morphine in incremental does up to 0.5 mg/kg or diazepam 0.1 mg/kg) or general anaesthesia may be required; a non-depolarizing muscle relaxant (atracurium 0.5–0.7 mg/kg or pancuronium 0.07–0.15 mg/kg) is preferable but succinylcholine (suxamethonium) (2 mg/kg) can be used safely up to 24 hours post-burn.[34–36]

If possible, the vocal cords should be visualized so that subsequent decisions about converting the translaryngeal tube to a tracheotomy can be made on the basis of the degree of original laryngeal injury.[20] The tube calibre must be the largest possible to facilitate tracheal toilet. The tube must be secured with straps or tape that encircle the patient's head above and below the ears.[22,37] The magnitude of facial swelling should be anticipated so that the endotracheal tube is not cut so short the outer end disappears when this occurs. The endotracheal tube must be uncuffed in children younger than 2 or under 20 kg; in adults, a high-volume, low-pressure tube must be used or the tube cuff should be inflated to minimum levels consistent with adequate ventilation and protection against aspiration even allowing a slight leak.[20,34] These precautions are taken to prevent tracheal damage which is not unusual in these patients who are often haemodynamically unstable (marginal perfusion of tracheal mucosa) and impossible to restrain (exaggerated mechanical trauma). Occasionally, it may be necessary to intubate the trachea with a fibreoptic bronchoscope over which an endotracheal tube has been sleeved; once the fibreoptic instrument is correctly positioned the endotracheal tube can be advanced blindly.[34,38] A cricothyrotomy is the method of choice for securing the airway if intubation is not possible[22,39] because of the difficulties and hazards of doing tracheostomies as an emergency in unintubated burn victims.[20] Decisions about how long to leave the endotracheal tube in place are complex and need to be individualized. They must be based on considerations of the patient's status, the patient's prognosis, the requirement for operations, the presence of uncontrolled pulmonary infection, the degree of respiratory failure, the severity of laryngeal injury, the duration of intubation, and the realization that a tracheostomy done in optimal circumstances does not increase the morbidity or mortality of burn victims.[20,40]

Respiratory failure

A pulmonary parenchymal injury reflected by impaired oxygenation often does not become clinically apparent until 24 hours or more after smoke exposure. When manifest earlier, the patient often has some pre-existing pulmonary compromise, has been exposed to especially toxic smoke from plastic compounds,[41] or has a significant burn injury. Patients with marginal oxygenation who fail to improve rapidly must be treated because alveolar volume loss and total atelectasis is such a prominent feature of this illness;[42] it is easier to prevent alveolar collapse than it is to restore alveolar volume to atelectatic pulmonary parenchyma.[43] The treatment is respiratory support with a volume-cycled ventilator using a relatively large tidal volume (12–15 ml/kg) and a synchronized intermittent mandatory mode of assistance so that the patient's respiratory muscles maintain some activity and monotonous tidal respiration is avoided. PEEP is often required; it must be used with awareness of its ability to impede venous return and thus limit cardiac output.[44] A pulmonary artery catheter may be needed to optimize fluid replacement when PEEP levels higher than 10 or 12 cm H_2O are needed. An effort must be made to keep the inspired oxygen concentration (FiO_2) below 0.55 to avoid oxygen toxicity.[45] Humidification of inspired gases, endotracheal suctioning, oral hygiene, exercise, optimal nutrition, and position changes remain critical components in the care of the intubated patient. When patients cannot tolerate the ventilator, systemic paralysis with a long-acting non-depolarizing agent (pancuronium or atracurium) may be required. Occasionally, conventional ventilators will not ventilate these patients adequately due to extreme decreases in compliance and mucous plugs or pneumonia. Resort to high-frequency jet ventilation may be successful in tiding patients over this stage of their illness; however, experience with this kind of respiratory assistance is limited.[46]

Carbon monoxide intoxication

As mentioned earlier, elevated levels of CoHgb must be presumed in fire victims and treated with 100% oxygen which reduces the elimination half-life of carbon monoxide to 60 minutes or less from 250 minutes when breathing air.[15] Elimination of carbon monoxide depends on the law of mass action so alveolar PO_2 is the critical factor in its removal rather than alveolar ventilation.[22] Compensatory and adaptive responses in intact organisms preclude the development of cellular toxicity during acute carbon monoxide poisoning which means that treatment needs to focus on rapid elimination only.[47] The debate over hyperbaric oxygen treatment to prevent or improve the neurological sequelae of carbon monoxide intoxication is ongoing.[48,49] As hyperbaric chambers are rarely available and hyperbaric treatment rarely results in neurological recovery, their use will be considered only rarely.[22]

Cyanide poisoning

Although it is clear that lethal levels of cyanide are measurable in burn victims of fires involving polymeric materials,[50] its precise importance in the mortality and morbidity of patients alive when they reach the hospital remains uncertain. Symptoms are non-specific; the diagnosis must be considered in patients who are slow to respond to treatment with persistent metabolic acidosis and elevated venous oxygen content. Although specific antidotes are available, treatment requires care and involves risks of hypotension and excessive levels of methaemoglobin formation.[25,51]

The burn wound

Specific treatment of the burn wound in the victim of smoke inhalation should be virtually ignored until the patient has demonstrated substantial cardio-respiratory stability. Once this has been achieved however, meticulous wound care with adequate pain control becomes of primary importance. It is clear that the burn wound has an adverse effect on pulmonary function which extends beyond the resuscitative period even in the absence of burn wound infection.[52,53] With infection, the lung is often the first visceral organ to herald multiple organ failure by developing some form of the adult respiratory distress syndrome.[54] The presence of smoke inhalation clearly renders the lung more vulnerable to the stresses provided by the burn wound per se, as well as the burn illness in general.[8] Patients with no burn do not have this added risk factor and experience a correspondingly lower mortality rate after smoke inhalation. Escharotomies must be done on full-thickness chest wall burns to limit restriction of chest wall movement with ventilation. These are usually not required before the oedema resulting from resuscitation forms underneath the unyielding eschar. Mafenide acetate (sulfamylon) would be a poor choice of topical wound agent in these patients because of the metabolic acidosis it causes due to carbonic anhydrase inhibition which often leads to severe hyperventilation.

Excision and grafting of the burn wound has the potential to eliminate the parietal source of infection and its adverse effect on pulmonary function. It will also shorten the period of the illness during which the lung is especially vulnerable to the many stresses coincident with wound care. It must be undertaken with extreme caution in patients who have a severe inhalation injury but is helpful for many provided the stresses of operation (pain, heat loss, blood loss) and anaesthesia can be controlled.[55,56] The strategy of excising and grafting a burn of the neck prior to converting an endotracheal tube to a tracheostomy does much to limit the mechanical and infectious complications associated with that form of airway access done through a burn wound.[20]

Glucocorticoids

Steroids do not modify the pathophysiological responses to smoke inhalation.[57] They do not help maintain the airway or limit the inflammatory response in a clinically detectable way in patients without a burn[58] and are associated with increased infection and mortality rates in patients with both an inhalation injury and a burn.[1] They should rarely, if ever, be used in the acute phase of the illness; perhaps to limit bronchospasm in patients known to be dependent on exogenous steroids.[22]

Antibiotics

Antibacterial drugs must be used carefully with full awareness of their adverse effect on mammalian cells and the potential they offer for the selection of resistant organisms. The consensus seems to be that prophylactic use of broad spectrum drugs offers little benefit although this assumption has not been tested rigorously. They may be of benefit in patients with significant polymicrobial bronchial infection prior to injury.

Future developments

As the state of the art for treating patients with inhalation injuries depends entirely on supportive measures, the potential for future developments would seem to be wide open. Even though our understanding of the inflammatory mediators which orchestrate respiratory insufficiency following smoke inhalation and burns is increasing rapidly,[52–54] this understanding does not equate with a specific effective therapeutic or prophylactic intervention. The purpose of attempts to define the sequence of cellular events responsible for the critical pathophysiological alteration following smoke inhalation is to identify a site in the inflammatory cascade at which an intervention might be helpful. Caution is necessary in this regard. It is doubtful if modification or inhibition of mediators detectable in serum, urine, or lymph will be effective; witness the failure of plasma exchange to alter the ultimate outcome of the illness. To be useful clinically, any such intervention must operate specifically at the site of mediator generation without disrupting homeostatic mechanisms at uninvolved tissue sites. With this general warning in mind, it is possible that surfactant replacement or topical administration of oxygen-free radical scavengers might prove useful.[33]

Although the treatment of inhalation injury is based on supportive measures useful in managing respiratory insufficiency of other aetiologies, the care of patients with an inhalation injury and a burn is complex and requires a comprehensive, integrated approach to all aspects of the illness which may last 2 to 3 weeks in a critical stage. It is best co-ordinated by a single experienced individual; a committee approach to the management of these patients is often disastrous. Patients with only smoke inhalation usually have an acute illness of one or two days duration, after which they rapidly approach their pre-injury status.[20] The interventions discussed in this chapter can be carefully withdrawn as the patient improves. It is best not to hurry this process allowing patients to consolidate their gains in a series of sequential steps. Serious long-term sequelae in smoke inhalation victims are unusual. They require comprehensive diagnostic efforts including lung biopsy to identify those patients with progressive pulmonary fibrosis or 'bronchiolitis obliterans' who may benefit from steroids or other forms of treatment designed to modulate the collagen in fibrous tissue.

Summary

Inhalation injury presents with a wide range of injury severity; it is characterized by diagnostic uncertainty in a sizable proportion of patients. Early patient management depends on the clinical status of the patient, not in an arbitrary way, on the presence or absence of the diagnosis alone. The insidious onset of relentless respiratory failure, after the compensations required to maintain adequate ventilation have exhausted the patient, can be mitigated by early aggressive treatment.

The presence of a significant burn increases the severity of any inhalation injury by several orders of magnitude.

References

1 Moylan JA, Chan C. Inhalation injury – An increasing problem. *Ann Surg* 1978; **188**:347.
2 *Fire and Smoke: Understanding the Hazards.* Committee on Fire Toxicology, Board on Environmental Studies and Toxicology. Commission of Life Sciences National Research Council. *National Academy Press,* 1986.
3 Clark WR, Nieman GF. Smoke inhalation. *Burns* 1988; **14**:473.
4 Traber DL, Herndon DN. Pathophysiology of smoke inhalation. In: *Respiratory Injury: Smoke Inhalation and Burns,* Haponik ER, Munster AM (eds). pp 61, McGraw-Hill, Inc., New York, NY, 1990.
5 Zawacki BE, Jung RC, Joyce J, Rincon E. Smoke, burns, and the natural history of inhalation injury in fire victims: A correlation of experimental and clinical data. *Ann Surg* 1977; **185**:100.
6 Herndon DN, Thompson PB, Brown M *et al.* Diagnosis pathophysiology and treatment of inhalation injury. In: *The Art and Science of Burn Care,* Boswick JA (ed), pp 153, Rockville, Aspen, 1987.
7 Levine MS, Radford EP. Fire victims: Medical outcomes and demographic characteristics. *Am J. Public Health* 1977; **67**:1077.
8 Clark WR, Bonaventura M, Myers W. Smoke inhalation and airway management at a regional burn unit: 1975–1983. Part I: Diagnosis and consequences of smoke inhalation. *J Burn Care & Rehabil* 1989; **10**:52.
9 Haponik ER, Summer WR. Respiratory complications in burns patients: Pathogenesis and spectrum of inhalation injury. *J Crit Care* 1987; **2**:49.
10 Demling RH, Lalond C, Liu Y, Zhu D. The lung inflammatory response to thermal injury: relationship between physiologic and histologic changes. *Surgery* 1989; **106**:52.
11 Haponik EF, Summer WR. Respiratory complications in burn patients: Diagnosis and management of inhalation injury. *J Crit Care* 1987; **2**:121.
12 Haponik ER, Munster AM. Diagnosis, impact, and classification of inhalation injury. In: *Respiratory Injury,* Haponik ER, Munster AM, (eds). pp 17, Smoke inhalation and Burns, McGraw-Hill, Inc., NY, 1990.
13 Heimbach D. Inhalation injury. In: *Burns of the Head and Neck,* Watchel TL, Frank DM (eds). pp 15, Major Problems in Clinical Surgery, Vol 29. W.B. Saunders, Philadelphia, PA. 1984.
14 Cahalane M, Demling RH. Early respiratory abnormalities from smoke inhalation. *J Am Med Assn* 1984; **251**:771.
15 Winter FM, Miller JN. Carbon monoxide poisoning. *J Am Med Assn* 1976; **236**:502.
16 Lee JM, O'Connell DJ. The plain chest radiograph after acute smoke inhalation. *Clin Radiol* 1988; **39**:33.
17 Shirani KZ, Pruitt BA, Mason AD. The influence of inhalation injury and pneumonia on burn mortality. *Ann Surg* 1987; **205**:82.
18 Head JM. Inhalation injury in burns. *Am J Surg* 1980; **139**:503.
19 Bingham HG, Gallagher TJ, Powell MD. Early bronchoscopy as a predictor of ventilatory support for burned patients. *J Trauma* 1987; **27**:1286.

20 Clark WR, Bonaventura M, Myers W, Kellman R. Smoke inhalation and airway management at a regional burn unit: 1974–1983. Part II: Airway management. *J Burn Care & Rehabil* 1990; **11**:121.

21 Dyer RF, Esch VH. Polyvinyl chloride toxicity in fires; hydrogen chloride toxicity in fire fighters. *J Am Med Assn* 1976; **235**:393.

22 Sharar SR, Heimbach DM, Hudson LD. Management of inhalation injury in patients with and without burns. In: *Respiratory Injury: Smoke Inhalation and Burns*, Haponik EF, Munster AM, (eds). pp 195, McGraw-Hill, Inc., New York, NY, 1990.

23 Covelli HD, Nessan VJ, Tutle WK. Oxygen derived variables in acute respiratory failure. *Crit Care Med* 1983; **1**:646.

24 Venus B, Matsuda T, Copiozo JB, Mathew M. Prophylactic intubation and continuous positive airway pressure in the management of inhalation injury in burn victims. *Crit Care Med* 1981; **9**:519.

25 Vogel SN, Sultan TR. Cyanide poisoning. *Clin Toxicol* 1981; **18**:367.

26 Barker SJ, Tremper KK. The effect of carbon monoxide on pulse oximetry and transcutaneous PO_2. *Anaesthesiology* 1987; **66**:677.

27 Ralston AC, Webb RK, Runciman WB. Potential errors in pulse oximetry. *Anaesthesia* 1991; **46**:291–5.

28 Vegfors M, Lennmarken C. Carboxyhaemoglinaemia and pulse oximetry. *Br J Anaesth* 1991; **66**:625–6.

29 Navar PD, Saffle JR, Warden GD. Effect of inhalation injury on fluid resuscitation requirements after thermal injury. *Am J Surg* 1985; **150**:716.

30 Scheulen JJ, Munster AM. The Parkland formula in patient with burns and inhalation injury. *J Trauma* 1982; **22**:869.

31 Herndon DN, Traber DL, Traber LD. The effect of resuscitation on inhalation injury. *Surgery* 1986; **100**:248.

32 Clark WR, Nieman GF, Goyette D *et al*. Effects of crystalloid on lung fluid balance after smoke inhalation. *Ann Surg* 1988; **208**:56.

33 Desai MH, Brown M, Micak R *et al*. Nebulization treatment of smoke inhalation injury in sheep model with dimethylsulfoxide, heparin combination and N- acetylcysteine. *Crit Care Med* 1986; **14**:321.

34 Goudsouzian N, Szfelbein SK. Management of upper airway following burns. In: *Acute Management of the Burned Patient*, Martyn JAJ (ed). pp 46, W.B. Saunders, Philadelphia, PA, 1990.

35 Shana PJ, Brown RL, Kirksey T *et al*. Succinylcholine induced hyperkalemia in burned patients – I. *Anesth Analg* 1969; **48**:764.

36 Martyn JAS, Goldhill DR, Goudsouzian NG. Clinical pharmacology of muscle relaxants in patients with burns. *J Clin Pharmacol* 1986; **26**:680.

37 Gordon MD, Ed. Burn care protocols: Anchoring endotracheal tubes on patients with facial burns. *J Burn Care & Rehabil* 1987; **8**:233.

38 Tan WC, Lee ST, Lee CN, Wang S. The role of fiberoptic bronchoscopy in the management of respiratory burns. *Ann Acad Med* 1985; **14**:430.

39 Toye FJ, Weinstein JD. Clinical experience with percutanous tracheostomy and cricothyroidotomy in 100 patients. *J Trauma* 1986; **26**:1034.

40 Hunt SL, Purdue GF, Gumming T. Is tracheostomy warranted in the burn patient? Indications and complications. *J Burn Care & Rehabil* 1986; **7**:492.

41 Davies JWL. Toxic chemicals versus lung tissue – an aspect of inhalation injury revisited. *J Burn Care & Rehabil* 1986; **7**:213.

42 Nieman GF, Clark WR, Wax SD *et al*. The effect of smoke inhalation on pulmonary surfactant. *Ann Surg* 1980; **191**:171.

43 Weisman IM, Rinaldo JE, Rogers RM. Positive end-expiratory pressure in adult respiratory failure. *N Eng J Med* 1982; **307**:1381.

44 Luce JM. The cardiovascular effects of mechanical ventilation and positive end-expiratory pressure. *J Am Med Assn* 1984; **252**:807.

45 Davis WB, Rennard SI, Bitterman PB *et al.* Pulmonary oxygen toxicity: Early reversible changes in human alvoelar structures induced by hyperoxia. *N Eng J Med* 1983; **309**:878.

46 Cioffi WG, Graves TA, McManus WF, Pruitt BA. High-frequency percussive ventilation in patients with inhalation injury. *J Trauma* 1989; **29**:350.

47 Halebian P, Robinson N, Barie P, Goodwin C, Shires GT. Whole body oxygen ventilation during acute carbon monoxide poisoning and isocapenic nitrogen hypoxia. *J Trauma* 1986; **26**:110.

48 Myers RA, Snyder SK, Enohoff TA. Subacute sequelae of carbon monoxide poisoning. *Ann Emerg Med* 1985; **14**:1163.

49 Grube BJ, Marvin JA, Heimbach DM. Therapeutic hyperbaric oxygen: Help or hindrance in burn patients with carbon monoxide poisoning. *J Burn Care & Rehabil* 1988; **9**:249.

50 Silverman SH, Purdue GF, Hunt SL, Bost RD. Cyanide toxicity in burned patients. *J Trauma* 1988; **28**:171.

51 Hall AH, Rumack BH. Clinical toxicology of cyanide. *Ann Emerg Med* 1986; **15**:1067.

52 Demling RH, LaLonde C. Systemic lipid peroxidation and inflammation induced by thermal injury persists into the post-resuscitation period. *J Trauma* 1990; **30**:69.

53 Demling RH, LaLonde C. *Burn Trauma*. Thieme Medical Publishers, Inc., New York, NY 1989.

54 Demling RH, Wenger H, LaLonde C *et al.* Endotoxin-induced prostanoid production by the burn wound can cause distant lung dysfunction. *Surgery* 1986; **99**:421.

55 Li-juan J, LaLonde C, Demling RH. Effect of anesthesia and positive pressure ventilation on early postburn hemodynamic instability. *J Trauma* 1986; **26**:26.

56 Engrav LH, Heimbach DM, Reus JL *et al.* Early excision and grafting vs. nonoperative treatment of burns of indeterminate depth: a randomized prospective study. *J Trauma* 1983; **23**:1001.

57 Nieman GF, Clark WR, Hakim T. Methylprednisolone does not protect the lung from inhalation injury. *Burns* 1991; **17**: 384.

58 Robinson NB, Hudson LD, Reim M *et al.* Steroid therapy following isolated smoke inhalation injury. *J Trauma* 1982; **22**:876.

6

Monitoring of the burn patient

R.J. KAGAN

Introduction

Advances in critical care monitoring have contributed significantly to the recent improvement in survival after major thermal injury. Monitoring of the burn patient is a complex process that involves all life support systems throughout the resuscitation and wound care phases of burn treatment. Specific therapeutic interventions are dictated by a multitude of clinical factors as well as the result of intensive, often sophisticated, monitoring.

Assessment of the burned patient during the acute care phase may require varying levels of monitoring on a continuous or intermittent basis. Young healthy patients with minor burn injuries may only require the occasional periodic assessment of vital signs, whereas those with greater risk factors will often demand a greater intensity of monitoring.

Monitoring must be both physiologically appropriate and clinically useful in the management of the burned patient. The importance of repeated bedside observations and evaluation cannot be overstated. Before utilizing the newer invasive modalities, one must weigh the risks and benefits of each monitoring method. Moreover, it is extremely important that the burn team develop a clinical protocol listing indications and techniques for obtaining certain physiological data.

Factors in assessing monitoring needs

A number of clinical factors must be considered when assessing monitoring needs in burned patients. These include burn size, inhalation injury, associated injuries, and pre-existing medical condition.

Burn size

Patients with minor burn injuries who present without additional complicating factors generally will not require admission to the Burn Unit for intensive care monitoring. Patients meeting the American Burn Association (ABA) Burn Center referral criteria[1] for moderate or major injury often develop large fluid shifts, haemodynamic instability, and alterations in biochemical status. Patients in this category generally require continuous monitoring of vital signs and hourly urine output as well as frequent laboratory determinations of serum electrolytes and arterial blood gases.

Inhalation injury

The presence of inhalation injury has a significant impact on morbidity and mortality in the burned patient.[2] This clinical syndrome is associated with an increased fluid requirement for resuscitation.[3] Patients with inhalation injury may require frequent blood gas determinations to monitor the adequacy of oxygenation and ventilation. Chest X-rays are only useful during the first 48 hours for the assessment of endotracheal tube placement and central venous catheter tip positioning as well as for ruling out the presence of pneumothorax, haemothorax, or atelectasis.

Associated injuries

Burn injuries may be accompanied by other forms of trauma; consequently, it is important to evaluate the patient for both known and unrecognized injuries as part of the initial assessment. Patients with associated injuries may require increased fluids and/or respiratory support. The level of monitoring must therefore be individualized based on the stability of the patient.

Underlying conditions

It is well documented that patients at the extremes of age ($<$2 or $>$60 years) have increased morbidity and mortality after thermal injury.[4-6] In addition, those patients with preexisting cardiac, pulmonary, metabolic, or renal disease are similarly less likely to tolerate the added stress of burn injury. This relates, in large part, to immune compromise and a lack of physiological reserve that is commonly seen when these conditions are present.

Cardiovascular monitoring

Non-invasive clinical methods

Heart rate, blood pressure, and electrocardiographic recordings are the primary modalities for monitoring cardiovascular status in any patient.

These parameters are generally sufficient to assess the physiological response of most burn patients during the phase of burn shock. Clinical interpretation of the data, however, should rely on the evaluation of trends rather than on isolated measurements.

Pulse rate

Patients with thermal injuries often present with tachycardia as a result of pain and hypovolaemia. In most patients, a heart rate (HR) greater than 120/min is usually an indication of hypovolaemia; however, pulse rate is a much less reliable indicator of hypovolaemia in the elderly patient due to the inability of the heart to increase its rate in response to a significant volume deficit. Heart rates below the normal range must be investigated thoroughly. With the exception of healthy, athletic patients, bradycardia may indicate the presence of hypoxaemia or cardiac failure, especially in the elderly and those with pre-existing cardiac disease.

Blood pressure

Blood pressure may be difficult to measure in the burned patient using standard sphygmomanometry, and is, at best, intermittent. Use of a small cuff tends to give falsely elevated readings. This is particularly true in children and large adults. In addition, because of the interstitial oedema that develops after burn injury, it may be difficult to auscultate the Korotkoff sounds. In this instance, it is often advantageous to utilize an ultrasonic Doppler device to obtain this data without using invasive techniques. The most common cause of hypotension in burn patients is hypovolaemia. This usually is preceded by tachycardia and may be due to fluid sequestration post-burn, associated injuries, or preexisting medical problems. Hypotension may also be due to depressed myocardial contractility, in which case invasive techniques are likely to be required. Hypertension is rare post-burn, most often being secondary to pain or a history of hypertension.

Electrocardiography

Although most young healthy burn patients rarely require monitoring of cardiac electrical activity, there are many instances where such monitoring is both helpful and necessary. Patients with pre-existing cardiac disease must be observed for primary arrhythmias, or those secondary to hypoxaemia, acidosis, or electrolyte imbalance. Although some controversy exists over the necessity for ECG monitoring of all patients with electrical injuries,[7,8] this is the only type of burn injury which can cause direct cardiac damage that resembles infarction. ECG monitoring may be difficult in patients with extensive burns of the torso and upper extremities; however, most topical agents are capable of conducting electrical impulses for monitoring. Needle electrodes or surgical staples may be helpful in the rare instance when surface leads cannot be maintained in contact with the skin. In ventilated patients, an oesophageal electrode system may be utilized.

Invasive methods

Haemodynamic monitoring utilizing invasive catheters has become widespread in most critical care units. These devices permit the direct, and sometimes continuous, measurement of arterial pressure, central venous pressure (CVP), and pulmonary vascular haemodynamics as well as the calculation of cardiac output, systemic vascular resistance, and oxygen consumption. The ability to measure these parameters must only be employed when routine treatment becomes ineffective, there is a history of preexisting cardiac disease, or there are complicating factors such as smoke inhalation or other life-threatening injuries.

Arterial blood pressure

The primary indications for direct arterial cannulation are the need for continuous monitoring of arterial pressure in the labile patient and the need for arterial access in patients with oxygenation difficulties (i.e. smoke inhalation, sepsis and respiratory distress syndrome). In the latter instance, it is generally prudent to place an indwelling cannula rather than risk arterial injury from multiple intermittent punctures. Arterial cannulae must be placed percutaneously, either directly or by Seldinger technique, through unburned skin under aseptic conditions. In all instances, the catheter must be secured to the skin and instrumentation properly calibrated. Although radial, femoral, or pedal arteries may be utilized, the location of the burn usually dictates the choice of insertion site. The most common complications of arterial cannulation are thrombosis, infection, and haemorrhage.[9] Arterial thrombosis is directly related to catheter composition and size, arterial diameter, and duration of catheterization. Ideally, catheters must be short and made of a Teflon material and preferably be 20-gauge or smaller. Thrombosis may lead to tissue ischaemia and possible loss of digits. Bacterial infection of an arterial catheter may occur although this is relatively rare. This complication can be avoided by strict adherence to protocols for changing cannulae and/or insertion sites every 48–72 hours. Lastly, bleeding is the most potentially lethal complication of arterial cannulation.[10] Exsanguination may occur quite rapidly if there is a disconnection in the tubing and if cardiac output is normal. All of the above complications can be minimized if one adheres to strict clinical guidelines for insertion and maintenance of these cannulae.

CVP monitoring

Central venous pressure serves as a measure of preload and may be helpful in assessing the adequacy of resuscitation during burn shock phase. Measurements can be obtained if the catheter tip is located in a major central vein. The absolute value of the CVP is not as important, however, as the change in response to therapy. CVP is generally safer and less expensive than pulmonary artery (PA) monitoring and many of the risks of pulmonary artery catheterization are avoided. The major disadvantage of this modality is its inability to reflect left heart preload in patients with preexisting pulmonary or cardiac disease.[10]

PA catheterization

The pulmonary artery catheter allows the measurement or calculation of CVP, pulmonary capillary wedge pressure (PCWP), cardiac output, and both systemic and pulmonary vascular resistance. Other calculable variables from PA catheterization which are often helpful in haemodynamic assessment and stabilization include arterio-venous oxygen difference and oxygen extraction ratio, shunt fraction, and estimation of the optimal positive end expiratory pressure (best-PEEP).

The Swan–Ganz catheter is most helpful in achieving maximal cardiac output and tissue oxygen delivery while minimizing pulmonary vascular congestion. It is possible to calculate left heart pre-load and cardiac afterload directly from PA catheter measurements; however, this information must be carefully interpreted. Patients with decreased preload will be benefited by increased fluid administration, while those with adequate left atrial filling pressures and decreased cardiac output will be best treated by the addition of inotropic drugs to the treatment regimen.

The primary use of PA catheters in burn patients is in the management of the patient who is difficult to resuscitate or the patient with sepsis. Difficulty in resuscitation is most often due to:

1. a delay in the initiation of intravenous therapy,
2. extensive burns,
3. deep burns,

4. the presence of inhalation injury, or
5. pre-existing cardiopulmonary disease.

When contemplating the placement of a PA catheter, one must weight the potential benefits against the inherent risks. This is particularly true in the burned patient in whom complications of invasive monitoring are increased significantly.[11] When choosing possible insertion sites, one must consider the potential complications associated with each method and weigh these against the personal experience of the treating physician.

Complications can generally be classified as mechanical or infectious.[12-14] Mechanical complications can be subdivided into those which occur early (pneumothorax, haemothorax, ventricular arrhythmias) and those which occur late (thrombosis and delayed haemorrhage). Infectious complications of indwelling central venous catheters are not as rare as once thought.[15,16] For this reason, it is wise to change the catheter site no less frequently than every 72 hours and minimize catheter repositioning.[15,17] Bacterial endocarditis and septic emboli have been reported in a significant number of patients with indwelling vascular catheters[18,19] and this complication is much more likely to occur in the critically ill burned patient.

Future of haemodynamic monitoring

Newer technologies for haemodynamic monitoring are emerging, including intravascular flow probes and electrodes,[20] and doppler imaging.[21] While more sophisticated invasive devices are being developed, it appears that continuous non-invasive monitoring modalities lacking many of the potential risks of catheter placement and maintenance will soon be available.[22,23]

Respiratory monitoring

Nearly all patients with major thermal injuries require the frequent monitoring of oxygenation, ventilation, and respiratory mechanics. Bedside clinical assessment can detect changes in airway patency, respiratory rate and effort, and breath sounds. Barring associated chest wall injuries, the most important initial tasks are the maintenance of an adequate airway and the recognition and treatment of carbon monoxide (CO) poisoning.

Clinical monitoring

Pulse oximetry and capnography have been proven to be useful non-invasive modalities to monitor oxygenation and ventilation respectively.[24] They permit the continuous appraisal of arterial oxygen saturation and end-tidal carbon dioxide content, while obviating the need for arterial puncture or cannulation. Serial chest X-rays should be obtained for the early detection of atelectasis, pneumonia, adult respiratory distress syndrome (ARDS), and evidence of barotrauma (pneumothorax, interstitial emphysema, and pneumopericardium).

Invasive monitoring

Patients with smoke inhalation or chest wall injuries often require mechanical ventilatory support. Although the non-invasive methods listed above may be applicable in these more seriously ill patients, invasive monitoring is frequently necessary. Carboxyhaemoglobin (CoHgb) levels are important in the early management of patients who have sustained their injuries in an enclosed space.[25] In particular, it is important to document that CoHgb is returning to normal levels with supplemental oxygen.[26] These levels must be obtained at the time of arterial blood gas sampling since a normal pO_2 does not preclude the presence of carbon monoxide poisoning. Serial blood gases via an indwelling arterial cannula are mandatory in monitoring of the adequacy of oxygenation and ventilation.

Ventilated patients also require the monitoring of respiratory mechanics, including peak inspiratory and mean airway pressure, dynamic compliance, and ventilator settings such as PEEP, tidal volume, and ventilatory rate. Close monitoring of these variables can provide the earliest clues to the onset of atelectasis, ARDS, or iatrogenic barotrauma. In addition, all tracheally intubated patients must have frequent microbiological surveillance of the respiratory flora in the event that pulmonary sepsis develops.

Monitoring of fluid balance and renal function

Clinical parameters

Fluid balance in the burned patient is best monitored by following urine output and body weight changes. Body weight increases most rapidly during the first 24 hours post-burn secondary to intravenous fluid administration. By the fourth to fifth post-burn day, much of this fluid is mobilized and body weight returns toward pre-burn values. Following this period of massive fluid shifts, daily weights are extremely helpful in assessing body water balance. This is particularly important because of the increased evaporative water loss that occurs following the destruction of the integumentary barrier.[27] Intake and output are the most essential clinical parameters monitored during burn shock resuscitation. These values must be recorded hourly during the acute phase of care.

Invasive parameters

A urinary catheter is required in nearly all patients requiring intravenous fluid resuscitation. Because urine output reflects vital organ perfusion, it must be maintained at 0.5 to 1.0 ml/kg/h. Care must be taken to assure that urine production is not the result of an osmotic diuresis since the rate of urine output is critical to the management of fluid replacement. Deep burns involving the muscle tissue may cause myoglobinuria or haemoglobinuria.[28] When a dark, port-wine colour of urine is detected, intravenous fluids must be increased in order to achieve a urinary output of 1.5 ml/kg/h. Alkalinization of the urine and the administration of an osmotic diuretic can minimize renal tubular damage.[29]

Because extraordinary volumes of fluid and electrolytes are administered both initially and throughout the course of burn care, it is also crucial to monitor serum electrolytes, glucose, BUN, and creatinine. This is particularly important when hypertonic solutions are used for resuscitation. Serum sodium values >160 mEq/l signal the existence of a hypertonic state which must be treated by altering the type and quantity of intravenous fluids being administered.[30] The additional monitoring of blood pH and base deficit are important in determining acid–base balance throughout the acute phase of burn care. Laboratory values must be repeated regularly during the day in all critically ill burn patients.

Metabolic and nutritional monitoring

Energy expenditure and protein metabolism are markedly increased following thermal injury. The metabolic rate may approach twice that in the resting uninjured state. This is largely due to an increase in catecholamine secretion which is mediated by the hypothalamus.[31] Numerous formulae have been proposed to estimate the calorie needs of the burned patient; however, indirect calorimetry provides a more accurate assessment of energy needs.[32] It is important that energy and protein requirements be reassessed throughout the hospital course as wound healing progresses.

In order to monitor the appropriateness of the nutritional support regimen, a number of clinical and laboratory parameters must be monitored regularly. Daily weights must be obtained in all burn patients in order to evaluate both the state of hydration and the maintenance of lean body mass. Calculations of dietary calorie and nitrogen intake must be performed to assure that metabolic needs are being met via the selected nutritional support regimen. In addition, laboratory evaluation of BUN, 24-hour urine urea nitrogen (and therefore nitrogen balance), blood glucose, hepatic function, and acute phase proteins (albumin, transferrin, and pre-albumin) are helpful to determine the adequacy of diet and to detect metabolic abnormalities secondary to underfeeding or overfeeding.

Gastrointestinal tract monitoring

Gastrointestinal bleeding from Curling's ulceration, once common in severely burned patients, is rarely a problem today. This is most likely due to the introduction of H_2-antagonists, earlier initiation of enteral nutritional support, and a more aggressive surgical approach to the burn wound. Yet, patients with burns in excess of 30% TBSA remain at relatively high risk for the development of gastroduodenal erosions or ulcerations.[33] For this reason, it is important to monitor gastric pH and titrate antacid prophylaxis. If a nasogastric tube is not in place, serial evaluation of haematocrit and stool guaiac or faecal blood must be performed regularly in the high-risk patient.

Bowel motility disturbances are also quite common after burn injury. Following the resolution of the ileus that often accompanies burn shock, it is also necessary to monitor enteric residuals via a nasogastric tube or the feeding tube. Abdominal girth and stool frequency must also be noted. Patients may develop a sudden intolerance to oral or enteral feeding, either as ileus or diarrhoea, secondary to underlying sepsis. Both of these conditions may be accompanied by large fluid losses, consequently care must be taken to search for clinical and laboratory signs of dehydration.

Bacteriological monitoring and infection

Infection and sepsis pose a serious threat to the survival of the thermally injured patient.[34] Treatment protocols must define the regular bacteriological monitoring of the burn wound. The avascular nature of the burn wound makes it an ideal medium for the growth of endogenous and exogenous bacteria which may penetrate the eschar and invade the underlying viable tissue. There must also be a regular clinical surveillance of the upper respiratory and lower urinary tracts for signs and symptoms of infection.

Clinical monitoring of infection

The burn wound must be examined at least once daily in order to detect infection at the earliest possible time and initiate appropriate treatment. Local signs of wound infection include:

1. conversion of partial thickness wounds to full-thickness,
2. focal or generalized discoloration of the burn wound,
3. rapid eschar separation, and
4. discoloration of the unburned skin at the wound margins.

Tracheally intubated patients and those with inhalation injuries must be examined for changes in auscultatory findings as well as the quality and quantity of pulmonary secretions. Patients with indwelling bladder catheters must also be evaluated for symptoms of lower urinary tract infection and the appearance of any urine sediment.

Laboratory evaluation

In patients with minor burns, twice weekly cultures of the wound surface may be adequate; however, patients with more extensive or deeper burns may also require serial quantitative biopsies to identify the predominant organism.[35] Histological examination of tissue is necessary in order to make a diagnosis of invasive burn wound sepsis. Sputum gram stains, culture and sensitivity patterns, and chest X-rays must be performed daily in all intubated patients as well as those with inhalation injury. Similarly, urinalysis and urine cultures must be obtained twice weekly in all catheterized patients.

Although there is no one parameter that will clearly allow one to make a diagnosis of sepsis, there are a number of clinical and laboratory findings that should be evaluated in high-risk patients. Clinical signs of sepsis include:

1. hypothermia,
2. altered mental status,
3. the sudden onset of ileus or diarrhoea,

    4. increased fluid requirements, or

    5. respiratory insufficiency.

Since burn patients are hypermetabolic and often hyperthermic, temperature elevation may not be a reliable diagnostic finding. Laboratory data that often precede these clinical findings include:

    1. thrombocytopaenia,

    2. metabolic acidosis,

    3. hypoxaemia, and

    4. glucose intolerance.

Blood cultures must be drawn based on clinical and laboratory findings as well as on a high index of suspicion; however, culture reports are often not available for 24 to 48 hours and may yield false negative results.[36] Therefore, the decision to initiate antibiotic treatment, fluid resuscitation, and/or pulmonary support must be based on an analysis of clinical and laboratory trends, rather than an isolated finding.

Monitoring of tissue perfusion

The burn wound

Monitoring of the burn wound for tissue perfusion and the level of demarcation is often difficult, even for the most experienced clinician. Careful serial observation of wound appearance and sensation are vital to the assessment of the depth of injury. This is particularly true for electrical injuries where demarcation of the extent of tissue necrosis may take 3 to 5 days. Newer non-invasive modalities, such as the laser Doppler,[37] may assist in the earlier diagnosis of depth of injury.

Subeschar compartments

Careful monitoring of the circulatory status of the extremities with full-thickness burns is necessary during the initial period of fluid resuscitation. As interstitial oedema forms beneath the inelastic eschar, tissue pressure may exceed capillary and arteriolar pressures to impair the flow of nutrients to the viable tissue beneath and distal to the eschar. Clinical parameters that must be examined include:

    1. cyanosis,

    2. delayed capillary filling,

3. diminished Doppler pulses, and
4. progressive neurological findings.

Since physical examination can be misleading, one must measure subeschar and/or subfascial pressure[38] utilizing an 18-gauge needle attached to a pressure transducer. A value of >30 mm Hg is significant and generally warrants the performance of an escharotomy and/or fasciotomy. It is also important to monitor compartment pressure in unburned extremities in those patients with extensive injuries and those in whom large volumes are required for resuscitation,[39] since permanent neurological sequelae have been reported in extremities that are distant from the site of burn injury. Subeschar and subfascial pressure measurements must be performed regularly, even after escharotomy, until tissue oedema has reached its maximum. Circumferential full-thickness burns of the chest can limit chest wall excursion and impair ventilation. This may be difficult to evaluate by physical examination alone and may be substantiated by the measurement of pCO_2 and inspiratory pressure. Expedient chest wall escharotomy can promptly alleviate this problem.

Summary

Monitoring of the burn patient has become more sophisticated as newer technologies have evolved. The future of critical care monitoring will most likely integrate newer continuous, non-invasive monitoring devices with computer systems that will not only record data, but also predict trends and initiate therapeutic feedback mechanisms. However, it is important to remember that not all patients will require the use of these newer techniques. While patients with major burn injuries may require invasive monitoring, those with minor injuries may only require the monitoring of basic clinical and laboratory parameters.

References

1 American Burn Association. Hospital and prehospital resources for optimal care of patients with burn injury: Guidelines for development and operation of burn centers. *J Burn Care & Rehabil* 1990; **11**:97.
2 Clark WR, Bonaventura M, Myers W. Smoke inhalation and airway management at a regional burn unit: 1974–1983. Part I: Diagnosis and consequences of smoke inhalation. *J Burn Care & Rehabil* 1989; **10**:52.
3 Deitch EA, Clothier J. Burns in the elderly. *J Trauma* 1983; **23**:891.
4 Navar PD, Saffle JR, Warden GD. Effect of inhalation injury on fluid resuscitation requirements after thermal injury. *Am J Surg* 1985; **150**:716.
5 Herd BM, Herd AN, Tanner NSB. Burns to the elderly – A reappraisal. *Br J Plast Surg* 1987; **40**:279.

6 Housinger T, Saffle J, Ward S *et al.* Conservative approach to the elderly patient with burns. *Am J Surg* 1984; **148**:817.

7 Purdue GF, Hunt JL. Electrocardiograph monitoring after electrical injury: necessity or luxury? *J Trauma* 1986; **26**:166.

8 Housinger TA, Green L, Shahangian S *et al.* A prospective study of myocardial damage in electrical injuries. *J Trauma* 1985; **25**:122.

9 Gauer PK, Downs JB. Complications of arterial catheterization. *Respir Care* 1982; **27**:435.

10 Pierson DJ, Hudson LD. Monitoring haemodynamics in the critically ill. *Med Clin N Am* 1983; **67**:1343.

11 Ehrie M, Morgan A, Moore FD *et al.* Endocarditis with the indwelling balloon tipped pulmonary catheter in burn patients. *J Trauma* 1978; **18**:664.

12 Kaye WE, Dublin HG. Vascular cannulation. In *Critical Care.* p 221. Civetta JM, Taylor RW, and Kirby RR, (eds). J.B. Lippincott, Philadelphia, PA. 1988.

13 Elliott CG, Zimmerman GA, Clemmer TP. Complications of pulmonary artery catheterization in the care of critically ill patients – a prospective study. *Chest* 1979; **76**:647.

14 McDaniel DD, Stone JG, Faltas AN *et al.* Catheter-induced pulmonary artery haemorrhage. *J Thorac Cardiovasc Surg* 1981; **82**:1.

15 Applefield JJ, Caruthers TE, Reno DJ *et al.* Assessment of the sterility of long-term cardiac catheterization using the thermodilution Swan–Ganz catheter. *Chest* 1978; **74**:477.

16 Sise MM, Hollingsworth P, Brimon JE *et al.* Complications of the flow-directed pulmonary artery catheter: A prospective analysis in 219 patients. *Crit Care Med* 1981; **9**:315.

17 Kaye W, Wheaton M, Potter-Bynoe G. Radial and pulmonary artery catheter related sepsis. *Crit Care Med* 1983; **11**:249.

18 Pinilla MC, Ross DF, Martin T *et al.* Study of the incidence of intravascular catheter infection and associated septicaemia in critically ill patients. *Crit Care Med* 1983; **1**:21.

19 Rowley K, Clubb KS, Smith GJ *et al.* Right-sided endocarditis as a consequence of flow-directed pulmonary artery catheterization. *N Eng J Med* 1984; **311**:1152.

20 Fabri PJ. Monitoring of the burn patient. *Clin Plast Surg* 1986; **13**:21.

21 Singer M, Clarke J, Bennett ED. Continuous haemodynamic monitoring by oesophageal doppler. *Crit Care Med* 1989; **5**:447.

22 Bernstein DP. Continuous noninvasive real-time monitoring of stroke volume and cardiac output by thoracic electrical bioimpedance. *Crit Care Med* 1986; **14**:898.

23 Shoemaker WC, Appel PL, Kram HB *et al.* Multicomponent noninvasive physiologic monitoring of circulatory function. *Crit Care Med* 1988; **16**:482.

24 Shapiro BA, Cane RD. Blood gas monitoring. Yesterday, today, and tomorrow. *Crit Care Med* 1989; **17**:573.

25 Zawacki BE, Jung RC, Joyce J *et al.* Smoke, burns and the natural history of inhalation injury in fire victims: a correlation of experimental and clinical data. *Ann Surg* 1977; **185**:100.

26 Winter FM, Miller JN. Carbon monoxide poisoning. *J Am Med Assn* 1976; **236**:1502.

27 Moncrief JA. Replacement Therapy. In: *Burns; A Team Approach*, p 169. Artz CA, Moncrief JA, and Pruitt BA Jr (eds). WB Saunders, Philadelphia, PA. 1979.

28 Walsh MB, Miller SB, Kugen LJ. Myoglobinemia in severely burned patients: Correlations with severity and survival. *J Trauma* 1982; **22**:6.

29 Eneas JF, Schoenfeld PY, Humphreys MH. The effect of infusion of mannitol–sodium bicarbonate on the clinical course of myoglobinuria. *Arch Intern Med* 1979; **139**:801.

30 Demling RH. Fluid replacement in burned patients. *Surg Clin N Am* 1987; **67**:15.

31 Wilmore DW. Catecholamines. Mediator of the hypermetabolic response to thermal injury. *Ann Surg* 1974; **186**:53.

32 Saffle JR, Medina E, Raymond J *et al.* Use of indirect calorimetry in the nutritional management of burned patients. *J Trauma* 1985; **25**:32.

33 Czaja AJ, McAlhany JC, Pruitt BA Jr. Acute gastroduodenal disease after thermal injury. An endoscopic evaluation of incidence in natural history. *N Eng J Med* 1974; **291**:925.

34 Alexander JW. The role of infection in the burn patient, p 103. In: *The Art and Science of Burn Care*. Boswick JA (ed). Aspen Publ., Rockville, MD, 1987.

35 Kim SH, Hubbard GB, McManus WF *et al.* Frozen section technique to evaluate early burn wound biopsy: A comparison with rapid section technique. *J Trauma* 1985; **25**:1134.

36 Marvin JA, Heck EL, Loebl EC *et al.* Usefulness of blood cultures in confirming septic complications in burn patients: evaluation of a new culture method. *J Trauma* 1975; **15**:657.

37 O'Reilly TJ, Spence RJ, Taylor RM *et al.* Laser doppler flowmetry evaluation of burn wound depth. *J Burn Care & Rehabil* 1989; **10**:1.

38 Saffle JR, Zeluff GR, Warden GD. Intramuscular pressure in the burned arm: measurement and response to escharotomy. *Am J Surg* 1980; **140**:825.

39 Kagan RJ, Waldbillig A, Merk T *et al.* The adequacy of escharotomy in the paediatric burn patient. (In preparation)

The paediatric burn patient

G.F. PURDUE, J.L. HUNT

Introduction

Burns in paediatric patients create many diagnostic and therapeutic problems not seen in adults. These include correct estimation of burn size and depth, fluid resuscitation and fluid maintenance, vascular access, airway management, nutritional support and prevention of sepsis. A child is not just a small adult, but a person who is even more devastated by the burn injury, and who is less able to respond to it.

Approximately one-third of burn unit admissions are children under the age of 15 years and one-third of all burn deaths involve children. Burns are second only to motor vehicle accidents as the leading causes of death in children older than one year. Most paediatric burns occur in the home and are very often the result of adult inattention or carelessness. However, about 10% are the result of deliberate abuse by adults.

Scald burns are the most common type of injury (50–60%), followed by flame burns (30%) and burns caused by contact with hot solids (10%). Chemical and electrical burns are very rare in children. Males predominate (about two-thirds), but this gender difference is not as large as in adults (75% male). Flame burns are frequently very severe; they often involve burning clothing, prolonged exposure and panic resulting in either flight or complete immobilization.

It is very difficult to make definitive statements based solely upon patient age, as any age groupings are also influenced by patient size and the other factors influencing burn severity. For this discussion, an infant is less than one year old, while a toddler is 1–3 years old. Because these children cannot talk or understand, burn team members must make special efforts to communicate at least daily (and sometimes more frequently, depending on injury severity) with their families.

Burn evaluation

Proper estimation of burn size is usually more difficult than in adults, yet the margin for error in a child is small. Accurate burn size determination is important because of its direct effect on resuscitation, surgical management and prognosis. The 'Rule of nines' does not apply to children because of their relatively larger head size and smaller lower limb size. As a rough rule, for each year under 10 years of age, 0.5% is subtracted from each lower limb and added to the head. The Lund–Browder and Berkow charts (see Chapter 2) divide the various body parts into smaller units (upper arm, lower arm, hand, etc) and make the appropriate correction for age.

Burn size estimation is most accurately performed by two people working as a team. One reads the relative percentages for each body part from the chart and records the result while the other person estimates the proportion of that body part burned. It is imperative that burn size and depth estimations be formally reviewed and updated on the second post-burn day, and again at a later date if necessary.

Child abuse must always be considered when treating or consulting on a burned child.[1,2] The pattern of burn injury is carefully evaluated with special attention paid to the presence of multiple burns (of the same or different ages), the presence or absence of splash marks, spared areas, bilateral symmetry ('stocking and glove') distribution, and well demarcated waterlines. The soles of the feet must always be inspected for the presence of any burn (even first degree). Non-burn trauma such as bruises, whip marks, fractures and head trauma are noted, and old medical records reviewed for prior injuries. If abuse is suspected, skull, chest and long bone radiographic series are obtained. The examiner must ask himself/herself the following questions:

Is the appearance, pattern and depth of burn consistent with the given history?

Does the given history remain constant with repeated telling?

When suspicion is aroused, the social worker and/or child welfare department must be contacted.

Burn depth is usually very difficult to estimate, especially in the early post-burn period. This is, in large part, due to the thinness of a child's skin. The depth of scald burns, especially in dark skinned infants, is notoriously difficult to estimate, and is frequently a degree deeper than originally appreciated. Underestimation of burn depth often occurs, even with experienced observers. Burn depth must be re-evaluated several times weekly to determine both prognosis and the need for surgical intervention.

Resuscitation

It is imperative that these small patients be kept warm.[3] All infants and those children with burns greater than 20% TBSA must have body temperature carefully monitored and maintained. Remember that the normal response to the burn is a resetting of core temperature upward to 38.5 °C to 39.0 °C. Never deliberately cool a burned child. Awareness of thermal maintenance must start at the scene of the burn injury and continue through the patient's entire hospital course. The first 24 hours after injury is especially important because of massive fluid infusions during resuscitation and the frequent opportunities for exposure (repeated burn evaluations, prolonged debridements, escharotomies and other procedures). The body surface area of a child relative to his mass is much greater than that of an adult while his ability to produce endogenous heat is much less. Thus minimal exposure to normal room temperature often produces a rapid and profound drop in core temperature. In addition, the infant under 6 months of age cannot shiver and must generate heat by non-shivering thermogenesis, whereby brown fat is catabolized under the influence of noradrenaline; an inefficient process. Maintenance of body temperature is best facilitated by a very warm environment with the additional use of an over bed warming shield and warming of intravenous fluids. Prolonged use of heating pads must be avoided because of the potential of conversion of back and posterior body burns to a deeper depth.

Burn resuscitation in the child is not an area where 'more is better', but neither is less. The margin between drowning a child and dehydrating him is a very small one. Fluid resuscitation requirements may be calculated by any number of different methods.[4-7] All achieve good results, but the key to success is familiarity. The Parkland formula is used: 4 ml Ringer's lactate (RL)/kilogram/% body surface area burned; one-half is given during the first 8 hours after injury and the rest in the next 16 hours. Several points should be made regarding the resuscitation of paediatric patients.

1. The patient must have a urinary catheter. The use of a urine bag or of weighed nappies (diapers) will not suffice. The child who requires resuscitation also requires meticulous monitoring of urine output.

2. In infants and toddlers with smaller burns, allowances must be made for non-burn daily maintenance fluids. In adults, the Parkland formula takes this non–burn requirement into account, but in children, maintenance fluids assume a significantly greater proportion of resuscitation than they do in adults.

    Example: 100 kg adult with a 50% burn.

    $4 \times 100 \times 50 = 20\,000$ ml. Non-burn maintenance is 2000–2500 ml or about 10% of the total amount.

    10 kg baby with a 50% burn. $4 \times 10 \times 50 = 2000$ ml.

    Non-burn maintenance is 1000 ml or 50% of the total amount. Begin resuscitation at the rate calculated by the Parkland formula and adjust upward by adding the maintenance fluids as necessary. Conversely, if the patient is able to drink fluids, intravenous infusion rates can be decreased. Adequate resuscitation is reflected by normal mentation, stable vital signs and a urine output of 1 ml/kg/h. During resuscitation, fluid rates are usually adjusted hourly to achieve proper urine volumes (half hourly if younger than one year).

3. Infants are very susceptible to hypoglycaemia, having limited glycogen reserves and little ability to carry out glucogenesis. Blood sugar is frequently monitored and glucose containing solutions added as necessary. Alternating or titrating RL and 5% dextrose in Ringer's lactate during the first day's resuscitation may be required to avoid either hypoglycaemia or hyperglycaemia.

4. Fresh frozen plasma (0.5 ml/kg/% burn) is started about 24 hours post-burn, just as in the adult, for burns greater than 20% TBSA. This is given at the same rate as the previous hour's fluids. When fresh frozen plasma is unavailable, aged plasma, heat sterilized plasma or albumin may be utilized.

5. After completion of resuscitation, fluid losses are replaced with dextrose 5% in 0.25% saline at 1.0 ml/kg/% burn rather than with dextrose 5% in water as in the adult. The use of this salt-containing solution helps minimize fluctuations in serum sodium which are aggravated by sodium-free solutions. In addition, the child must have the normal non-burn daily maintenance as dextrose 5% in 0.25% saline. The administration of glucose-free solutions must be avoided after the first 24 hours, especially in infants. The brain depends upon glucose just as it does upon oxygen for an energy substrate.[8] Clinical manifestations of

hypoglycaemia (<2.6 mmol/l) are an abnormal cry, listlessness or feeding difficulty. However, in the critically ill infant there is often no recognizable symptom complex. Diagnosis rests on a high index of suspicion and frequent blood glucose measurements.

6. A child younger than 2 years of age has a renal system best suited to conserving sodium.[9] This is reflected by an obligate free water loss (manifested by an inability to concentrate the urine) greater than expected. Ideally, urine output should be maintained as close as possible to 1 ml/kg/h.

It cannot be overemphasized that the fluid volume determined by a burn formula is only the starting point of the resuscitation. Exact volumes must be individually adjusted based on clinical response. An infusion pump or a burette must be used to accurately deliver the intravenous fluids. All intravascular catheters must be securely sutured in place and the child adequately restrained to prevent accidental displacement. Careful attention to detail during the resuscitation phase will ensure optimal results in the paediatric patient.

Respiratory management[10–13]

The respiratory mechanics of the young child are very different from those of the adult. The newborn infant is an obligate nose breather, a characteristic which permits breathing while feeding. Children have poorly developed intercostal and diaphragmatic muscles and are primarily abdominal breathers. Hence, abdominal distention is very poorly tolerated. Care must be taken to ensure that nasogastric tubes are properly functioning at all times. Respiratory rate will vary with age and activity, but a rate >40 is definitely abnormal.

The most common cause of acute bradycardia in a burn patient is hypoxia. Corrective steps must be taken immediately. Start by increasing inspired oxygen concentration to 100% and work rapidly through the causes of hypoxia. If the appropriate size paediatric equipment is not available or when its function is questioned, fall back on the old standby of mouth-to-mouth or mouth-to-nose ventilation.

Children have proportionally more airway dead space than does an adult, with infants having a dead space in their nose and pharynx equal to one-half of their tidal volume. The increased work of breathing in a child may require earlier intubation and ventilation than would be expected of an adult. Paediatric endotracheal tubes and tracheostomy tubes have no cuff until the internal diameter reaches 5.0 mm. The size of these uncuffed tubes must be selected so that ventilation to 30 mm Hg peak pressure can be achieved. As a general rule, this size is the same as the tip of the patient's fifth finger or the width of their nares or may be calculated using the formula:

Tube size = (16 + age) divided by 4.

A starting place for tube selection is given in Table 7.1.[9] These tube sizes are smaller than those normally recommended because of the airway swelling frequently seen in burned children. Initially, there may be a small air leak which seals with progressive oedema. When intubating a child, always have endotracheal tubes one size larger and one size smaller than that recommended. Nasotracheal intubation is the method of choice. This route stents the tube, preventing kinks, and is better tolerated, permitting food and oral toilet while preventing the patient from chewing on the tube. The straight blade laryngoscope must be used during intubation if direct visualization is necessary. A difficult intubation may be aided by the use of a fibre-optic bronchoscope. Intubate a child when you think of it, waiting will jeopardize its survival.

Table 7.1. *Endotracheal tube diameter*

Age	Tube size (I.D.)
0–6 mo	3.0 mm
7–12 mo	3.5 mm
1–2 yr	4.0 mm
3–4 yr	5.0 mm
5–8 yr	5.5 mm

Adequate fixation of the endotracheal tube is absolutely essential and may be life-saving. In infants the difference between being tracheally intubated and being extubated is a matter of millimetres. Unfortunately, the burned face makes fixation of the tube extremely difficult. The close proximity of topical burn wound agents, continual changes in size of the face and neck (due to burn oedema), and the fluid exuding through a facial burn often cause failure of the usual methods of fixation. Careful fixation utilizes a safety pin through the side of the tube (but not occluding the lumen), then secured with an umbilical tape passed around the head.

Patented fixation devices may be very helpful, although pressure necrosis of soft tissue must be avoided. An endotracheal tube is very easily dislodged and is often difficult or impossible to re-insert. In the latter instance tracheostomy performed as an emergency may be life-saving, but its performance is usually technically difficult.

The small internal diameter of paediatric endotracheal tubes increases the risk of obstruction by secretions. Special attention must be paid to adequate suctioning of the tube, especially when first admitted as the patient often does not receive adequate pulmonary toilet during transport or while in the emergency room. During the early post-burn period, tracheal secretions are often very viscous and may contain carbonaceous particles and pieces of mucous membranes. Endotracheal suctioning is facilitated by instilling normal saline rather than acetylcysteine, which may cause bronchospasm in children.

Tracheostomy in the child may be considered at an earlier date than in the adult, i.e. in the first week. Inadvertent endotracheal tube dislodgement frequently occurs and the long endotracheal tube length makes suctioning difficult; both of which are obviated by tracheostomy. The 'unable to be reintubated' situation must always be kept in mind. Improved pulmonary toilet can be achieved, as can better oral toilet, an important factor in avoiding oral candidiasis. The smaller dead space and lower resistance of the tracheostomy contribute to better pulmonary mechanics. These factors along with an increased incidence of subglottic stenosis produced by prolonged endotracheal intubation, must be balanced against the increased risk of bronchopneumonia and late complications such as tracheal stenosis, created by a tracheostomy. In some cases, tracheostomy may be required in children who cannot be extubated because of persistent upper airway obstruction despite steroids and racemic adrenaline. Children may be discharged with the tracheostomy tube in place.

Circulation[14-16]

The resting pulse of children is higher than that of adults, generally increasing with decreasing age from 70 as an adolescent, to 100 as a preschool child to 140 for the crying newborn. Blood pressure is initially equal in the arms and legs, until 1 year of age when systolic pressures in the legs increase to about 40 more than the arms. Diastolic blood pressures are usually equal in the arms and legs. Normal blood pressure values are given in Table 7.2.

Table 7.2. *Normal blood pressure values*

Age	Systolic/Diastolic
Newborn	60–90 /30–60
1 year	65–120/50–70
3 years	75–125/45–90

The use of the correct size blood pressure cuff is necessary to ensure accurate measurements. The cuff must cover two-thirds of the upper arm of the child.

Transfusion of 1–1.5 ml/kg of packed red blood cells will increase haematocrit by 1 and can be given at a rate of 10–15 ml/kg/h in the absence of haemorrhage or shock. Colloid replacement may be performed with 25% albumin (1 ml/kg) for albumin levels less than 2.0 gm/dl in order to maintain intravascular oncotic pressure.

Vascular access[17]

Intravascular access is often a major problem in the paediatric burn patient because of the distribution of the burn wound, the presence of subcutaneous oedema, and the need to change catheters every 72 hours to minimize catheter sepsis and suppurative thrombophlebitis. The number of cutdown sites is obviously limited and in burn patients these often become infected and may be a nidus for septic thrombophlebitis. While interosseous infusions provide emergency vascular access, usage is necessarily short term. The femoral vessels provide an excellent route of access when other avenues fail. The catheter should be no larger than 19 gauge and the use of the femoral route is avoided during the first 24 hours post-burn because of the increased risk of arterial occlusion during this period. Despite dire warnings from paediatricians to the contrary, in a burned child the femoral route is easily obtained and associated with minimal complications. In the authors' unit ninety-five children, ranging in age from 1 month to 14 years, had 564 femoral catheters with only 4 complications. There were 471 venous and 93 arterial catheters. All complications were vascular. The only two patients with limb threatening arterial occlusion were profoundly hypotensive at the time of cannulation. There were no septic complications and no growth discrepancies in any patients with a maximum follow-up of 8 years.

Wound management

Silver sulphadiazine (Flamazine BP; Silvadine USP) is the usual agent of choice for burn wound care. It is very well tolerated with few metabolic complications. Less than 0.5% of patients exhibit allergic symptoms, and, while leucopaenia may occur, it is transient and corrects despite continued use of this agent.[18] The open technique of wound care is usually preferred, but special care must be taken with children to ensure that all burned areas are adequately and continuously covered with the topical agent, to prevent desiccation and conversion of the burn to a deeper depth. If continued complete coverage is a problem (or if the child eats silvadine), then a closed occlusive dressing technique is used.

Immersion of a child with a large burn in water during debridement is contra-indicated, as hyponatraemia may occur rapidly. Early surgical excision and showering rather than immersing patients has minimized this problem. Hexachlorophene (Phisohex R) soaps are contra-indicated in burned children because of the potential of neurological damage and seizures. Chlorhexidine (Hibiclens R) provides a safe, effective means of cleansing burn wounds when diluted half and half with water. Peripheral circulation in limbs with circumferential constricting eschar must be carefully and frequently monitored. Vascular compromise occurs earlier than in an adult and may occur following a deep partial thickness circumferential burn. Escharotomy technique is the same as in the adult.

Burn wound excision and grafting are frequently done later than would be done in adults, unless the wound is definitely full thickness. The thin skin of a child contributes to the difficulty of clinically distinguishing various depths of partial thickness from full thickness injuries while the mechanical limitations of wound excision and proportionally deeper donor sites also promote a more conservative approach to wounds of indeterminate depth than for comparable burns in the adult.

Nutritional support

Special attention is always directed to the maintenance of adequate nutrition because of the very limited nutritional reserve of the child. While enteral feeding is much preferred, there must be no hesitation to begin parenteral hyper-alimentation early in the patient's course (second post-burn day) or when there is any sign of intolerance (diarrhoea, dehydration and hypernatraemia) to oral feeding. While mother's milk is ideal, in practice, this is rarely a satisfactory option in the intensive care setting because of the involved logistics. Oral and tube feedings are begun as soon as the postburn ileus resolves. Prepared formulae may be used for children younger than 1 year while a high-protein high-calorie diet or ready prepared one calorie/ml feedings are used for older children. Tube feedings will usually be required in patients with burns >25% TBSA. Pre-operative orders for children must minimize the nil by mouth period. Tube feedings may often be continued up until 4 hours prior to surgery. Glucose containing solutions must be given intravenously during any fasting periods.

Serum sodium levels are monitored daily as wide fluctuations occur and significant symptoms, such as seizures, occur at higher levels (about 125 mmol/l) than in the adult. Children must be denied free access to water in order to prevent a psychogenic water drinking syndrome.

Sepsis

Burn wound sepsis may occur earlier (2–4 days) and at lower colony counts ($>10^3$ per gram of eschar) than in the adult. The infant especially, has a defective immune system which appears to have little recognition and defence against a variety of organisms, especially gram positive cocci. However, prophylactic antibiotics are no longer utilized. Routine burn wound cultures and quantitative biopsies must be performed (usually one culture per 15% TBSA). Culture results of moderate or $>10^3$ colony count in an infant with a burn >20% TBSA or a pre-school child >40% TBSA are treated with appropriate antibiotics.

The febrile response of the burned child can be very misleading. Children may manifest a temperature up to 40 °C as a response to the burn injury itself. Generally, this phenomenon first occurs within 24 hours of the injury and continues as daily (often nightly) temperature spikes until the wound is nearly closed. Before accepting this as the cause of fever, other aetiologies of fever must be ruled out. Otitis media is relatively common (7% of burn patients less than 4 years old), and must be high in the differential diagnosis of fever. Meningitis is extremely rare (two cases in 1200 consecutive paediatric burn patients) and is usually accompanied by neurological signs. If CNS infection is suspected, a spinal tap must never be performed through or in near proximity to the burn. A cisternal tap is required in children with back burns.

Persistent hypothermia and/or increased sensitivity to cooling after the first post-burn day are ominous signs of sepsis. The minimum daily temperature must be watched as closely as the maximum temperature. In a clinically ill child, a normal or low WBC with 'lymphocytosis' often indicates profound bacterial sepsis in which the majority of 'lymphocytes' are found to be very immature neutrophils when the specimen is hand counted.

Early diagnosis of sepsis requires a high index of suspicion as the signs are very subtle. The nurse's statement that 'Johnny doesn't look right today' is often the first indication of sepsis. Clinical deterioration in a child is often much more rapid than in the adult, so suspicion of sepsis must be rapidly acted upon. The minimum therapeutic response includes intravenous access and urinary catheter insertion and administration of intravenous antibiotics to cover either the patient's known wound flora or bacteria endemic in the burn unit at that time.

Oral candidiasis (thrush) is a frequent opportunistic organism in paediatric burn patients, sometimes causing major problems with oral hygiene and nutrition. In addition, children are able to absorb candida from the gastrointestinal tract (persorption), resulting in systemic sepsis. Oral nystatin is given to all children with major burns. Candida septicaemia may present in the early post-burn period as a monomicrobial infection which must be treated with amphotericin B. Candida cultured simultaneously from any two organ systems and is also an indication for systemic amphotericin therapy. If amphotericin is not tolerated, fluconazole may be tried.

Burns are tetanus prone wounds. Tetanus can occur despite partial tetanus immunization. Both tetanus hyperimmune globulin and tetanus toxoid must be given on admission when the patient is not fully immunized.

Complications

Hypothermia is a preventable complication which may have profound systemic effects. The haemoglobin/oxygen dissociation curve is shifted to the left, blood flow to the skin is decreased and the metabolic rate is increased. Each degree centigrade drop in core temperature requires approximately a 16% increase in metabolic rate to return temperature to normal. Remember that 'normal' in the burn patient is >38 °C. The patient must also be kept warm in the operating room. This must include warming the room pre-operatively with maintenance at 29–32 °C and 30–50% relative humidity. A heating blanket is used under the patient and all fluids used both internally and externally are warmed. An external overhead infrared heater is often necessary. If the surgical team is not uncomfortably warm, the room is too cold. Efforts must be made to expose as little skin area as possible and all body areas not directly involved in the procedure must be kept covered. Hypothermia delays clotting, increases acidosis and may lead to later rebound hyperthermia with vasodilation, hypovolaemia and shock; a fatal event if not recognized and treated promptly.

Acute gastric dilatation may be a significant problem (especially during transport) if adequate nasogastric suction is not established and maintained. This complication may easily lead to respiratory compromise, vomiting and aspiration.

Hypertension[19,20] is an idiopathic response to a large burn, which has been reported to occur in up to 20% of children with large burns. Onset is gradual, often beginning weeks after the injury and continuing through the early recovery period, after which it nearly always disappears. While hypertension may be manifested by irritability, crying and rubbing or banging of the head, it is usually asymptomatic. Treatment is with hydrazaline, reserpine or alpha methyldopa depending upon severity.

Curling's ulcer[21] is a stress response originally described in children. It, along with haemorrhagic gastritis was once quite common, but the use of anti-ulcer prophylaxis with either antacids or H_2 blockers have made perforation and significant bleeding very rare.

Superior mesenteric artery syndrome, obstruction of the third portion of the duodenum by the superior mesenteric artery, is a rare complication in this era of nutritional awareness. Occurrence usually follows a large weight loss. It is manifested by persistent post-prandial vomiting of bilious material, although continuous feedings may be well tolerated. Diagnosis is made with an upper gastrointestinal series of X-rays with contrast media showing obstruction of the duodenum, relieved by placing the patient in the prone position.

Summary

The burned child presents special problems in management. Events occur more rapidly and the margins for error are smaller than in the adult. Attention to detail is paramount in achieving an optimal result.

References

1 Purdue GF, Hunt JL. Child abuse – An index of suspicion. *J Trauma* 1988; **28**:221.
2 Lenoski EF, Hunter KA. Specific patterns of inflicted burn injuries. *J Trauma* 1977; **17**:842.

3 Klaus M, Fanaroff A, Martin RJ. The physical environment. In: *Care of the High Risk Neonate*, pp 94–112. WB Saunders, Philadelphia, PA, 1979.

4 Carvajal HF. A physiologic approach to fluid therapy in severely burned children. *Surg Gyn Obst* 1980; **150**:379–84.

5 Herndon DN, Curreri PW, Abston S, Rutan TC, *et al*. Treatment of burns. *Curr Prob Surg* 1987; **29**:347–9.

6 Bowser-Wallace BH, Caldwell FT Jr. A prospective analysis of hypertonic lactated saline v. Ringer's lactate–colloid for the resuscitation of severely burned children. *Burns* 1986; **12**:402–9.

7 O'Neil JA. Fluid resuscitation in the burned child – A re-appraisal. *J Ped Surg* 1982; **17**:604–7.

8 Volpe JJ. Hypoglycaemia and brain injury. In: *Neurology of the Newborn. Major Prob Clin Ped* 1981; **22**:301–20.

9 Wilkinson AD. Some aspects of renal function in the newly born. *J Ped Surg* 1973; **8**:103–16.

10 Persky MS: Airway management and post-intubation sequelae. In: *Critical Care Pediatrics*, pp 10–15. Zimmmerman SS, Gildea JH (eds). WB Saunders, Philadelphia, PA, 1985.

11 Strong RM, Passey V. Endotracheal intubation: Complications in neonates. *Arch Otolarynol* 1977; **103**:329–335.

12 Calhoun KH, Deskin RW, McCracken MS, *et al*. Long- term airway sequelae in a pediatric burn population. *Laryngoscope* 1988; **98**:721–25.

13 Fearon B, Ellis D. The management of long term airway problems in infants and children. *Ann Otol* 1971; **80**:670–7.

14 Levin DL, Morriss FC, Moore GC. Normal blood pressures for various ages. Appendix C. In: *A Practical Guide to Pediatric Intensive Care*, p 652. Levin DL, Morriss FC, Moore GC (eds). Mosby, St. Louis, Missouri, 1984.

15 Horan MJ. Task force on blood pressure control in children: Report of the second task force on blood pressure control in children – 1987. *Pediatrics* 1987; **79**:1–25.

16 Malavade V, Gorman JG, Abebe LS. Component transfusion therapy. In: *Critical Care Pediatrics*, pp 112–124. Zimmerman SS, Gildea JH (eds). WB Saunders, Philadelphia, PA, 1985.

17 Iserson KV, Criss E. Intraosseous infusions: A usable technique. *Am J Emerg Med* 1986; **4**:540–2.

18 Thomson PD, Moore NP, Rice TL *et al*. Leucopenia in acute thermal injury: evidence against topical silversulfadiazine as the causative agent. *J Burn Care & Rehabil* 1989; **10**:418–20.

19 Akrami C, Falkner B, Gould AB *et al*. Plasma renin and occurrence hypertension in children with burn injuries. *J Trauma* 1980; **20**:130–4.

20 Notterman DA. Hypertension. In: *Critical Care Pediatrics*, pp 10–15. Zimmerman SS, Gildea JH (eds). WB Saunders, Philadelphia, PA. 1985.

21 McAlhany JC, Czaja AJ, Pruitt BA. Antacid control of complications from acute gastroduodenal disease after burns. *J Trauma* 1976; **16**:645–9.

8

Nutrition

M.A. MARANO, M.R. MADDEN,
J.L. FINKELSTEIN, C.W. GOODWIN

Introduction

The importance of nutritional support in the management of critically ill
trauma and/or burned patients is well accepted. Nutritional support is a
prerequisite for survival following major burn injuries; however, many
questions regarding optimal nutrition in critically ill man remain un-
answered and warrant further investigation. Major burn injury presents
unique nutritional problems as a result of extreme hypermetabolism and
an increased demand for energy-yielding substrates.

The goal

The overall goal of administering nutritional support to critically ill
burned patients is to improve survival as well as to decrease associated
morbidity. In order to accomplish this goal, nutritional support must
minimize the erosion of lean body mass effectively and help to maintain
immunocompetence. Loss of vital protein stores, a process referred to as
'auto-cannibalization', often occurs following major burn injury, as
metabolic demands are usually greater than the available energy (calorie)
supplies. Additional factors which increase metabolic demands include
infections and associated traumatic injuries. An unmatched metabolic
demand will eventually result in protein-calorie malnutrition, cachexia,
weight loss and an increased morbidity and mortality. By contrast, the
administration of nutritional support may result in closely matched
caloric supply and demand, thereby improving survival.

Hypermetabolism

The victims of major burns are always at risk from nutritional deficiencies
because of an exaggerated and prolonged hypermetabolic state. There is

Table 8.1. *Important clinical factors correlated with post-burn hypermetabolism*

Size of surface burn	Inhalation injury
Systemic sepsis	Body temperature
Ambient temperature	Activity level
Dressing changes	Thermogenic effect of feeding
Timing of wound closure	Surgical procedures

a continued demand for additional protein and total calories during this period. Cuthbertson[1] first described the metabolic consequences of burn injury as an initial 'ebb' or hypometabolic phase (24–48 hours) and a subsequent 'flow' or hypermetabolic phase (after 48 hours). Others [2,3] have suggested a correlation between hypermetabolism and circulating 'stress' hormones such as catecholamines or circulating lipo-polysaccharide. Multiple other factors contribute to the increased energy needs of burned patients including environmental temperature, core body temperature, activity level, size of surface burns, the thermogenic effect of feeding, timing of wound closure, and presence of concurrent sepsis and/or inhalation injury[4] (Table 8.1). Attempts to decrease the hypermetabolic response following burn injury, in an attempt to prevent lean body mass erosion, have met with mixed success.[5,6] Presently, the benefit of ameliorating the post-burn hypermetabolic response remains unproven in a clinical setting as there has been no clear demonstration of a survival advantage in man.

Energy balance

The mainstay of a sound nutritional philosophy for the treatment of these injuries is to balance energy supply with demand. Standard practice has evolved towards providing critically ill burned patients with additional energy substrates, in the form of protein, lipid and carbohydrate, as well as micronutrients and vitamins. In order to support this practice as the central goal of nutritional support, one must understand the consequences of both inadequate and excessive delivery of calories.

Inadequate calories

Glucose derived from hepatic glycogen stores is used preferentially during stress and/or starvation. Eventually, gluconeogenic amino acids and fat stores are mobilized to meet additional energy needs. The clinical consequences of hypocaloric feeding were described by Bartlett who

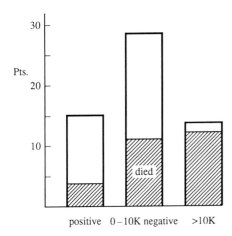

Fig. 8.1. Consequences of persistent underfeeding in a critically ill population. Cumulative caloric balance related to outcome (Bartlett *et al*).[7]

demonstrated that surgical patients with a cumulative kilocalorie deficit greater than 10 000 developed more complications and had a higher mortality rate compared with a similar control group[7] (Fig. 8.1). Additionally, there is recent evidence that immunosuppression following a major burn may be, in part, due to malnutrition and that aggressive and timely nutritional support may improve immune function.[8–11]

Excessive calories

Nutritional support in excess of needs, particularly during administration of parenteral nutrition, may lead to pulmonary and hepatic dysfunction.[12,13] In patients with pre-existing pulmonary disease, overfeeding results in excessive CO_2 production which may contribute to prolonged ventilator dependency. Chronic carbohydrate overfeeding may also induce fatty infiltration of the liver indicated by an elevation of serum transaminases. Moreover, there is a lack of evidence that overfeeding is in anyway beneficial to patients even if pre-injury malnutrition were present.

Nutritional assessment and needs

Nutritional assessment

Major burn victims are at risk from developing nutritional deficiencies due to immobilization and inactivity, fever, infections and frequent gastrointestinal intolerance to oral feeding. Therefore, every burned patient must received a careful baseline nutritional assessment on admission in order to assess nutritional progress during the hospital stay. Because many standard nutritional assessment parameters have limited application following such an injury, monitoring progress is difficult and often inaccurate.

Ideally, a complete nutritional assessment includes detailed dietary history, the measurements of body weight and other anthropometric indices, nitrogen balance determinations and measurement of the level of plasma proteins.[14] The latter include plasma levels of albumin, pre-albumin, transferrin and retinol binding protein (RBP).[15] However, dietary history may be unavailable while measurements of body weight are often inaccurate owing to fluid resuscitation. In addition, measurement of other anthropometrics, such as triceps skin-fold thickness, may be impossible because of extremity burns and nitrogen balance is often inaccurate due to loss of nitrogen through surface burn wounds. Pre-resuscitation body weight is commonly used as a basis for estimating total caloric needs as reported in a recent survey of dietary practices in burn centres.[16] After mobilization of resuscitative fluids, serial body weight measurements may again become a reasonably acceptable means of monitoring nutritional progress. In addition, the most common method used to monitor caloric goal achievement is a daily calorie intake record. As there is no single best monitor of nutritional status, overall assessment is best made by analysing a variety of information.

Determining calorie needs

Total caloric needs may be estimated by several empirically derived formulae and measured at the bedside using the method of indirect calorimetry. The most commonly used formulae in the United States are the Curreri formula[17] and the Harris–Benedict formula modified for burn injury although other calculations are acceptable (Table 8.2). The Toronto formula is another empirically derived formula which takes into account caloric intake, body temperature and elapsed time since burn injury.[18] Adult formulae tend to overestimate paediatric requirements and are therefore inaccurate in children. As a result, several formulae have been derived specifically for the paediatric age group (Table 8.3).

Measurement of energy expenditure

An accurate assessment of total caloric need may be obtained by measuring energy expenditure. Energy expenditure measurements are

Table 8.2. *Commonly used adult formulae used to estimate total caloric requirements in burned patients*

1.	*Curreri formula:*
	25 kcal/kg + (40 kcal × %BSA burn)
2.	*Harris–Benedict formula* modified for burned patients:
	BEE × stress factor

Men: BEE = 66 + (13.7 × W) + (5.0 × H) − (6.8 × A) × stress factor
Women: BEE = 655 + (9.6 × W) + (1.8 × H) − (4.7 × A) × stress factor

%BSA burn	Stress factor
10%	1.4–1.6
10–20%	1.6–1.8
20–30%	1.8–1.9
30–40%	1.9–2.1
>40%	2.1–2.3
BEE =	basal energy expenditure
W =	weight in kilograms (kg);
H =	height in centimetres (cm);
A =	age in years (yr);
%BSA =	% body surface area burn for correlation with stress factor.

3.	*Toronto formula (TF)*
	TF = −4343 + (10.5 × %BSA) + (0.23 × CI) +
	(0.84 × BEE) + (114 × temp (°C)) −
	(4.5 × PBD)
	CI = calories received in previous 24 hours
	PBD = post-burn day

performed at the bedside using indirect calorimetry. Resting energy expenditure (REE) is determined from O_2 consumption and CO_2 production in a relationship as defined by the Weir equation. Compared with estimated calorie requirements from empirical formula calculations, indirect calorimetry measures energy needs and allows determinations of the respiratory quotient (RQ), defined by the ratio of CO_2 production to O_2 consumption. As defined by this relationship, an increase in the RQ from the typical fasting ratio of 0.70 to 0.85 towards 1.0 implies a net increase in CO_2 production, a by-product of carbohydrate metabolism, usually as a result of delivery of additional calories. Therefore, a low RQ during nutritional support may suggest inadequate total calorie delivery. Conversely, an RQ of about 1.0 suggests adequate carbohydrate feeding when considered with other nutritional assessment parameters.

There are several limitations to using indirect calorimetry. As measurements are valid only for the immediate time frame, serial measurements must be performed during the hospital stay to best

Table 8.3. *Commonly used paediatric formulae used to estimate total caloric requirements in burned patients*

1.	Calories appropriate for age and weight × stress factor			
	Age factor	*kcal/kg*	*TBSA burned*	*Stress*
	0–6 mo	115	10%	1.1
	6–12 mo	105	10–20%	1.1–1.2
	1–3 yr	100	20–30%	1.2–1.4
	4–6 yr	85	30–40%	1.4–1.5
	7–10 yr	86	>40%	1.5–1.7
	11–14 yr	60 (males)		
	15–18 yr	42		
	11–14 yr	48 (females)		
	15–17 yr	38		
2.	Modified Curreri 'Junior' formula <12 mo: 80 kcal/kg + (30 kcal × % BSA burn) 1–12 yr: 60 kcal/kg + (30 − 35 kcal × %BSA burn)			

approximate the changing needs of each patient. Additionally, factors which increase daily energy requirements above resting conditions must be considered in determining daily needs. Such 'stress factors' include surgical procedures, infection, increased activity levels and frequent dressing changes. A common empirical practice is to multiply the REE by a stress factor of 1.2 to 1.5 in order to achieve a stable body weight.

Energy expenditures are usually normalized to the square metre of body surface area and time ($kcal/m^2/h$) in order to allow comparisons between individuals. Total body surface area calculations are based on height and admitting (preresuscitation) weights.

Determining protein needs

Nitrogenous products are released in increased quantities via the urine and burn wounds during the hypermetabolic phase. During this catabolic period, delivery of total calories and the proportions of carbohydrate, fat and protein affect the net release of amino acids from the protein stores of skeletal muscle mass.

A commonly used expression of the relationship between total calories and protein (i.e. nitrogen) in a given nutritional formula is the calorie to nitrogen ratio (cal:N). A lower ratio signifies a higher proportion of nitrogen delivered per calorie. Although there is an ongoing debate regarding the optimal nitrogen requirements following burn injury,[8] some empirically derived guidelines for protein needs are presented:

> In patients with <30% TBSA burns, use a 150:1 formula:
> Grams of protein needed =
> Total caloric need × 0.143 divided by 4.
> In patients with >30% TBSA burns, use a 125:1 formula:
> Grams of protein needed =
> Total caloric need × 0.167 divided by 4.

Administration of nutritional support

Route of feeding

Nutritional support may be administered by various routes. In patients who are able to eat, an oral diet is the logical choice. However, most burned patients either cannot or will not eat enough to meet caloric goals without additional enteral or parenteral support. Enteral feeding may be administered into the stomach by an in-dwelling nasogastric tube, or into the small bowel by a naso-enteric tube or by a percutaneous jejunostomy feeding tube. Parenteral nutrition is administered through a centrally placed indwelling intravenous catheter, usually inserted via the subclavian vein or internal jugular vein. When standard 'polymeric' enteral formulae are not well tolerated, 'elemental' diets, consisting of amino acids and easily digestible carbohydrates, may be an alternative to parenteral nutrition.

Recent investigation has focused on the role of the gut mucosa in preventing translocation of bacteria and on a favourable immune benefit during enteral feeding.[19–21] Additionally, physical and metabolic complications due to enteral feeding are less common than with parenteral nutrition. Based on a growing body of scientific evidence demonstrating benefit for gastrointestinal feeding compared with parenteral nutrition, the general consensus is that oral or enteral feedings are preferable to parenteral nutrition whenever the gastrointestinal tract is functional. Parenteral nutrition is indicated when the gut is persistently nonfunctional due to ileus or intolerance for a period of at least several days. Moreover, there is no clinical benefit to parenteral nutrition unless it is continued for a minimum of 5 days. Finally, parenteral nutrition may be used as an adjunct to meet caloric needs when enteral feedings cannot alone meet the goals.

Complications of enteral and parenteral nutrition

The complications associated with enteral nutrition vary according to the methods and components used. Patients who have sustained major burn injuries will develop gastric stasis, typically lasting several days and often do not tolerate an oral diet. Similarly, attempts at nasogastric feeding are met with varied success. Patients with an altered level of consciousness, associated trauma or inhalation injury are more likely to aspirate gastric contents. Enteral feeding may be possible early after injury if radiological or endoscopy facilities are available to aid in the accurate placement of catheters into the small bowel. In such cases, a nasogastric tube is simultaneously placed to facilitate gastric decompression. The incidence of diarrhoea is approximately 30% in enterally fed burned patients and its aetiology is multifactorial. Recent investigation suggests that implementation of enteral feeding within 48 hours post-burn and limiting fat content (<20% of calories) may result in a decreased incidence of diarrhoea.[22] Other factors contributing to diarrhoea include faecal impaction, antibiotic use and lactose-containing diets. A recent survey details a commonly used approach to treat diarrhoea in this population.[16]

Administration of parenteral nutrition is associated with several well-described complications. Insertion of a central venous catheter, a prerequisite for total parenteral nutrition, may result in a pneumothorax. The incidence of this complication is related to the experience of the operator. All intravenous catheters as well as those used for parenteral nutrition administration, must be changed every 72 hours in order to minimize the incidence of catheter-related sepsis. Common metabolic complications include hyperglycaemia, an increase in serum transaminases, and essential fatty acid deficiency (EFAD). Because of these potential complications, as well as others, the use of parenteral nutrition is only justified when the benefits clearly outweigh the risks.

Mechanics of feeding

In adults, commercially available enteral feedings are initiated at full strength at a continuous rate of 30ml/h. During intragastric feeding, residual volumes are monitored every 4 hours. Retention of greater than 50% of delivered volume over 4 hours constitutes intolerance and therefore feedings are stopped until another trial is begun in 8 hours. The rate of feeding is increased in small increments over 24–48 hours until the desired target rate is achieved. Intragastric feeding may be withheld overnight prior to surgery to lessen the risk of aspiration upon induction of anaesthesia and to avoid uncontrolled diarrhoea during surgical excision and grafting procedures. Recent preliminary reports suggest that feeding patients by the nasogastric route during the immediate perioperative period may be accomplished safely. Enteral feeding may be stopped at any time without immediate complication.

In adults, parenteral nutrition is initiated at a continuous rate of 20–30 ml/h and the rate increased in small increments over 24–48 hours until the desired target rate is achieved. Frequent sampling of serum glucose levels is necessary as hyperglycaemia is common, due to the high concentration of dextrose in these formulations. Insulin may be added to parenteral solutions to control moderate hyperglycaemia. However, uncontrolled metabolic abnormalities preclude continued use. Lipids are administered simultaneously with continuous dextrose–amino acid solutions. Parenteral nutrition may be continued during surgical procedures if patients are metabolically stable. Cessation of parenteral nutrition is safely accomplished by serial reductions in the rate of infusion, 50% at any one time, over a period of 6 hours.

Timing of feeding

Aggressive nutritional support is often necessary for survival following a major burn. Therefore, the concepts of early and immediate feeding, particularly by the enteral route, have recently attracted much attention and are foci of ongoing investigations. The issue of potential benefits versus risks is pertinent in patients following burn injury. Those who believe in these concepts initiate immediate feeding within 12 hours of injury while early feeding is initiated by others within the first 36–48 hours.

The hypothesis that immediate feeding abates the post-burn hypermetabolic response has been supported experimentally.[5] However, evidence for clinical benefit is still lacking. Opponents to the philosophy of immediate feeding argue that the potential risk of aspiration outweighs unproven benefit especially during the early hypometabolic phase of injury. If immediate feeding is to be administered safely, direct enteral (jejunal) feeding is preferred with simultaneous gastric decompression.

There is a growing consensus among burn specialists in the United States that in selected patients, initiating enteral feeding during the early post-burn hypermetabolic period (24–48 h) is safe and beneficial particularly when gastric stasis has resolved. A judgment of safety must take into account the age of the patient, associated medical problems and surface burn area, as well as the need for surgical wound closure. As stated earlier, patients with a prolonged ileus will require either direct enteral feeding or parenteral nutrition.

Components (macronutrients)

Carbohydrates, lipids and proteins are the macronutrient substrates used as body fuel. As stated earlier, the goal of nutritional support is to balance energy supply and demand. However, calories derived from carbohydrate sources are metabolized differently than those from lipid sources. This concept was alluded to earlier during a discussion of optimal calorie to nitrogen ratios. A secondary goal of nutritional support is to provide a balance of macronutrients to minimize the lean body mass erosion often associated with post-burn catabolism.

Carbohydrates

Increased gluconeogenesis occurs in patients following burns and/or systemic sepsis.[23] The rationale for carbohydrate administration as an energy source is to attenuate 'auto-cannibalization' by reducing amino acid conversion to fuel via gluconeogenesis.

The ideal amount of enterally delivered carbohydrate calories is unknown; however, data from parenteral nutrition studies suggest an optimal glucose infusion rate of approximately 5 mg/kg/min (approximately 50% of total calories) is necessary to maximize protein sparing but avoid side effects. Potential side effects of carbohydrate overfeeding during nutritional support include fatty infiltration of the liver and prolonged ventilator dependency, since CO_2 production is a by-product of carbohydrate metabolism.[13,24] Regular determination of the respiratory quotient in such patients greatly facilitates planning the level of caloric support.

Protein

Cuthbertson demonstrated the association of negative nitrogen balance with trauma.[25] The mechanisms responsible for this observation are multifactorial. Contributing factors to net protein catabolism include inactivity during critical illness, the post-burn hypermetabolic response, intercurrent infections or systemic sepsis, a need for multiple surgical procedures and an inadequate supply of total calories and protein.

An important component of nutritional therapy is the supply of adequate dietary protein to reduce skeletal protein loss. Although there is general agreement regarding the importance of dietary protein, particularly to improve immune function, optimal protein requirements have not been determined in burns. Moreover, a reliable method for monitoring net protein balance is lacking in this population.

It is generally accepted by empirical observation that the rate of protein administration should be approximately 1.5 gm/kg/day and 2.0 to 2.5 gm/kg/day in the critically ill and in patients with major burns respectively.[8] Using these guidelines, approximately 20% of total daily energy needs will be due to dietary protein administration.

Lipid

Administration of lipids in nutritional support therapy has several beneficial effects. Lipids are a good source of calories and tend to decrease catabolism of endogenous proteins. Additionally, dietary lipid administration prevents essential fatty acid deficiency and is a carrier for fat soluble vitamins. As approximately 25% of CO_2 is produced from lipid oxidation, weaning a patient from prolonged mechanical ventilation occasionally may be facilitated by decreasing dietary carbohydrate and substituting with dietary lipid.

However, the focus of recent investigation is on potentially deleterious effects of currently available lipids on immune function following burn injury,[9,26] prompting a search for new lipid products with a variety of fatty acid components. The relatively high fat content of enteral preparations (up to 30% of total calories) may also contribute to intolerance manifested as diarrhoea.[22] On the other hand, the minimal amount of dietary lipid necessary to prevent essential fatty acid deficiency, usually associated with parenteral nutrition, is 1–2% of total calories.

Although the optimal requirements of proteins and lipids in patients with major burns remain unknown a high calorie, high protein oral diet is recommended. As most patients are unable to meet calorie requirements by the oral route alone, enteral and parenteral nutritional supplementation is commonly necessary. When using parenteral nutrition, the following calorie proportion guidelines are recommended, 65–80% carbohydrate, 15–20% protein, 5–15% lipid. Commercially available

Table 8.4. *Optimal composition of enteral and parenteral formulae (% total calories/day) for burned patients*

Carbohydrate	65–80%
Protein	15–20%
Lipid	5–15%

enteral products generally conform to the following total calorie proportions,[16] 50% carbohydrate, 20% protein and 30% lipid; however, optimal proportions for burned patients are similar to parenteral formulae guidelines (Table 8.4).

Micronutrients: trace minerals and vitamins

There is currently a lack of guidelines for trace mineral supplementation in the burned patient although there is some evidence that requirements parallel calorie and protein needs. In a recent survey of United States burn centre practice, patients were considered 'high risk' for trace mineral deficiency if they either had greater than 40% body surface burns or were receiving parenteral nutrition as the sole source of calories. Only in these sub-populations was specific trace mineral supplementation considered. The most common minerals supplemented were zinc, iron, copper, manganese and chromium.[27]

While the general nutritional consequences of the hypermetabolic state following major burn injuries are recognized, little is known about specific vitamin requirements. Under these circumstances, fat-soluble vitamins should be administered at recommended daily allowance (RDA) levels, while water-soluble vitamins may be increased with little potential for deleterious side effects.[15]

State of the art

Burned patients have benefited greatly from an improved understanding of the importance of nutritional support during critical illness. Reasonable methods of nutritional assessment and many commercially available products to meet specific needs are established. The importance of a high calorie, high protein diet is understood. As a result, morbidity and mortality rates have improved, at least in part, due to aggressive nutritional supplementation using both enteral and parenteral formulae.

Based on an improved understanding of the pathophysiology following burn injury, nutrients can be supplied better in effective amounts and complications minimized. Although understanding is far from complete, fewer burned patients succumb to malnutrition as a result of their injuries.

Future developments/areas of active research

At the current time, a number of new therapies are in various stages of investigation and development in an attempt to further improve the nutritional support of critically ill patients. In general, these potential therapies are either new components or nutritional adjuncts. Branched chain amino acids (BCAA) and glutamine are amino acid products being studied as enrichment formulae.[28–30] The goal of amino acid component therapy is to reduce protein catabolism during hypermetabolic periods. Lipid components under study include medium chain triglycerides and marine oils.[31,32] Medium chain triglycerides may be more efficiently utilized compared with other lipids. Marine oils are alternative body fuels which may also modify the host response to infection. Promising adjuncts to nutritional support include growth hormone and insulin-like growth factor (IGF–1) which may result in an improved net nitrogen balance and more rapid wound healing.[33] Finally, investigation regarding the host metabolic response to injury and sepsis may lead to therapies designed to reduce the nutritional demand following major burn injuries.

Further investigation is necessary for the future development of safe and effective nutritional products for use in critically ill patients, and specifically in major burn victims.

References

1 Cuthbertson DP. Post-shock metabolic response. *Lancet* 1942; **i**:433–7.
2 Marano MA, Fong Y, Barber A *et al.* Energy expenditure response to thermal injury, hormone background, and endotoxin/LPS in man. *Proc Am Burn Assn* 1989; **134**.
3 Wilmore DW, Long JM, Mason AD *et al.* Catecholamines: mediators of the hypermetabolic response to burn injury. *Ann Surg* 1974; **180**:653–70.
4 Allard JP, Jeejheebhoy KN, Whitwell J *et al.* Factors influencing energy expenditure in patients with burns. *J Trauma* 1988; **28(2)**:199–202.
5 Mochizuki H, Trocki O, Dominioni L *et al.* Mechanism of prevention of postburn hypermetabolism and catabolism by early enteral feeding. *Ann Surg* 1984; **200**:297–310.
6 Wood RH, Caldwell FT Jr., Bowser-Wallace BH. The effect of early feeding on postburn hypermetabolism. *J Trauma* 1988; **28**:177–83.

7 Bartlett RH, Dechert RE, Mault JR *et al.* Measurement of metabolism in multiple organ failure. *Surgery* 1982; **4**:771–9.

8 Alexander JW, Macmillan BG, Stinnett JD *et al.* Beneficial effects of aggressive protein feeding in severely burned children. *Ann Surg* 1980; **192**:505–17.

9 Alexander JW, Saito H, Ogle CK *et al.* The importance of lipid type in the diet after burn injury. *Ann Surg* 1986; **204(1)**:1–8.

10 Chandra S, Chandra RK. Nutritional regulation of the immune responses: basic considerations and practical applications. *J Burn Care & Rehabil* 1985; **6(2)**:174–8.

11 Forse RA. Nutritional effects on the immune response in surgical patients. *J Burn Care & Rehabil* 1985; **6(3)**:295–303.

12 Askanazi J, Rosenbaum S, Hyman A *et al.* Respiratory changes induced by the large glucose loads of total parenteral nutrition. *J Am Med Assn* 1980; **243**:1444–7.

13 Lowry S, Brennan M. Abnormal liver funtion during parenteral nutrition: relation to infusion excess. *J Surg Res* 1979; **26**:300.

14 Morath MA, Miller SF, Finley RK *et al.* Interpretation of nutritional parameters in burn patients. *J Burn Care & Rehabil* 1983; **4**:361.

15 Bell SJ, Wyatt J. Nutrition guidelines for burned patients. *J Am Diet Assn* 1986; **86(5)**:648–53.

16 Williamson J. Actual burn nutrition care practices: a national survey (part II). *J Burn Care & Rehabil* 1989; **10(2)**:185–94.

17 Curreri PW, Richmond D, Marvin J *et al.* Dietary requirments of patients with major burns. *J Am Diet Assn* 1974; **65**:415.

18 Allard JP, Pichard C, Hoshino E *et al.* Validation of a new formula for calculating the energy requirements of burn patients. *J Parenteral & Enteral Nutr* 1990; **14(2)**:115–18.

19 Alverdy J, Chi HS, Sheldon GF. The effect of parenteral nutrition on gastrointestinal immunity: the importance of enteral stimulation. *Ann Surg* 1985; **202**:681–4.

20 Deitch EA, Winterton J, Li M *et al.* The gut as a portal of entry for bacteraemia. *Ann Surg* 1987; **205**:681–92.

21 Saito H, Trocki O, Alexander JW *et al.* The effect of route of nutrient administration on the nutritional state, catabolic hormone secretion, and gut mucosal integrity after burn injury. *J Parenteral & Enteral Nutr* 1987; **11(1)**:1–7.

22 Gottschlich MM, Warden GD, Michel M *et al.* Diarrhoea in tube-fed burn patients: incidence, etiology, nutritional impact, and prevention. *J Parenteral & Enteral Nutr* 1988; **12(4)**:338–44.

23 Wolfe RR, Durkot MJ, Allsop JR *et al.* Glucose metabolism in severely burned patients. *Metabolism* 1979; **28**:1031–9.

24 Burke JF, Wolfe RR, Mullany CJ *et al.* Glucose requirements following burn injury: parameters of optimal glucose infusion and possible hepatic and respiratory abnormalities following excessive glucose intake. *Ann Surg* 1979; **190**:274–83.

25 Cuthbertson DP. Observation on the disturbance of metabolism produced by injury to the limbs. *Quart J Med* 1932; **1**:233–46.

26 Saito H, Trocki O, Heyd T *et al.* Effect of dietary unsaturated fatty acids and indomethacin on metabolism and survival after burn. *Proc Am Burn Assn* 1985; **17**.

27 Shippee RL, Wilson SW, King N. Trace mineral supplementation of burn patients: a national survey. *J Am Diet Assn* 1987; **87(3)**: 300–3.

28 Cerra FB, Upson D, Angelico R *et al.* Branched chain amino acids support postoperative protein synthesis. *Surgery* 1982: **92**:192–9.

29 Cerra F, Hirsch J, Mullen K, Luther W, Blackburn G. The effect of stress level, amino acid formula, and nitrogen dose on nitrogen retention in traumatic and septic stress. *Ann Surg* 1987; **205**:282–7.

30 Souba WW, Smith RJ, Wilmore DW. Glutamine metabolism by the intestinal tract. *J Parenteral & Enteral Nutr* 1985; **9(5)**:608–17.

31 Bach A, Babayan VK. Medium-chain triglycerides: an update. *Am J Clin Nutr* 1982; **36**:950–62.

32 Alexander JW, Saito H, Ogle CK, Trocki O. The importance of lipid type in the diet after burn injury. *Ann Surg* 1986; **204**:1–8.

33 Ziegler TR, Young LS, McK. Manson J, Wilmore DW. Metabolic effects of recombinant human growth hormone in patients receiving parenteral nutrition. *Ann Surg* 1988; **208**:6–16.

9

Infection in burn patients

C.G. WARD

Introduction

Though infections in burn patients are common and are the major cause of death, they are poorly understood. Believing infections are straight forward is to fail to appreciate their gravity and to be over-optimistic. There is more to an infection than identification of the causative agent and choosing a suitable antibiotic. They are complicated, insidious, incestuous, and intricate. Infections do not all occur in the same manner. Each is different in the way it gets started, how it progresses, and how it ends. There are three components to an infection: the host, the infecting organism, and the timing. In addition, each component has the elements of being qualitative, quantitative, and dynamic.

The skin has four major functions:

1. to keep heat inside the body,
2. to keep water inside the body,
3. to keep invading organisms outside the body, and
4. to give contour to the body.

Care for a burn victim is directed at restoring these functions. Of the four, keeping invading organisms under control is the most difficult to duplicate.

The immunological consequences of a burn are far reaching. Once the injury is larger than 10–15% total body surface area in size, the physiological impact is no longer local, but affects distant and systemic protective mechanisms.[1] Burn patients can have early infections from unusual circumstances, but usually become infected at 5–7 days post-injury.

In the beginning

Infecting agents originate from two locations, from inside or outside the body. Those from inside the body can come from several areas. As a consequence of the burn trauma, bacteria can spread systemically if not controlled by intrinsic or extrinsic mechanisms. Intrinsic bacteria can come from a localized abscess, an infected lung, a urinary tract infection, or the gut. The deranged immunological function that occurs as a consequence of the burn can release an otherwise controlled infection allowing it to progress and spread. A concern today is burn patients who have an established human immunodeficiency virus (HIV) infection. Their disease does not improve and burning can initiate a cascade of complications.

Extrinsic organisms

Infections originating from the outside come from two locations: the general environment and from the care givers. Infections from the environment may begin at the same time as the burn occurs. A patient burned in a boat explosion, for example, will instinctively and understandably jump into the surrounding water which is frequently contaminated. For practical, clinical reasons, the circumstances of all injuries must be known in order to anticipate mechanisms of wound contamination.

The care givers may contaminate a patient during the giving of care by spreading organisms originating from themselves or from one patient to another. No matter what the origin, it is ominous when a single organism is spread amongst many patients. Pasteur was aware, and others have demonstrated the effect of passage on the virulence of bacteria. As bacteria are passed from one animal to another there is a selection of the virulent form of an organism. In mice a lethal inoculum of *Pseudomonas aeruginosa* can be reduced from 100 000 organisms to less than ten bacteria.[2–4]

In the burn ward, there are times when a species of bacteria becomes common to several patients. This occurs because a resident organism contaminates several patients. Historically, such epidemics cause burn care facilities to be shut down. This has been true for *P. aeruginosa* in the past and is true for methicillin resistant *Staphylococcus aureus* (MRSA) today. A passage-like phenomenon occurs in the burn unit as the bacteria are passed from one patient to another and resistant forms of the organism are selected out.

People, and the equipment they use to care for burn patients, can be a source of infection. During transport to a hospital, a patient with a large burn will frequently have intravenous lines placed by transport personnel. These are done with the haste of an emergency and as life-saving manoeuvres. They are not, however, always done with the best of sterile techniques. Similar manoeuvres occur in the emergency room. Expediency is the priority. Intravenous lines placed under such conditions must be removed early.

A bottle of hand lotion used by several members of the burn team, once contaminated, becomes a reservoir of bacteria. Clothes that brush against an infected wound can carry organisms to a distant site. Hands unwashed are both historical and current causes for passing infections among patients. Food given to patients to improve and aid recovery can be dangerous. Fresh vegetables and fruits are contaminated with organisms and must be cooked before being given to susceptible patients. Equipment used to prepare purée diets can be a source of contamination. Ice machines harbour water-borne bacteria, particularly *P. aeruginosa*.[5,6] Standing water becomes easily contaminated. The water in which flowers are kept, even plant soil, harbours bacteria. None of these must be allowed in the burn centre. This policy also applies to non-patient areas, for a staff member can become contaminated and pass organisms around the unit. Contaminated equipment passed from one patient to another can convey bacteria, selecting a virulent form of the organism that begins to kill patients. Equipment such as intravenous and respiratory tubing, ventilation bags, instruments for dressing changes, bedding, rehabilitation equipment, even the rooms when they become unduly dirty must be changed frequently.[7] Still, bacteria hide in the most obvious but overlooked locations. Techniques must be in place at all times in a burn centre to prevent cross-contamination.

Intrinsic organisms

For potential sepsis and wound contamination, the patient is his own worst enemy. Flora from the gastrointestinal (GI) tract, the respiratory tree, the vagina, and the skin contaminate wounds. Burn wound dressings are changed in a variety of ways. Some are done in rooms designed exclusively for wound care. Others are changed at the time of bathing. Not all dressings, however, are done outside the patient's rooms; many are changed while the patient is in bed because the condition of the patient is critical. This is not the best condition, for the bedding and the contents of the room are always contaminated. A patient having bowel movements in bed is soiling his wounds continually. An intubated patient coughing up infected sputum continually inoculates his wounds and the endotracheal tube acts as a conduit for infecting the respiratory tree.

Though bacteria in the GI tract do not remain contained following major trauma to the host,[8–10] by using the GI tract normally for feeding, translocation of bacteria is diminished when compared to parenteral feeding. Parenteral feeding, without enteral feeding, promotes bacterial translocation from the gut.[11] The translocation of organisms is not limited to bacteria. In addition to spread from the vagina, infra-mammary folds, and the perineum, *Candida albicans* also moves from the GI tract.[12]

Normally, bacteria are in the GI tract in a symbiotic relationship with the body. It is frequently forgotten that bacteria in the gut are to the benefit of the body, but at the same time they are usually confined. It is when they get out in disproportionate numbers that problems begin. Normally they escape in small numbers and the body is able to tolerate and control them. Bacteraemia is associated with bowel movements and brushing of teeth, yet there is not an associated sepsis unless there are malfunctions in the primary protective mechanisms or anatomical defects are present. An immunologically compromised patient may not tolerate a daily bacteraemia; individuals with heart valve lesions are classically prone to endocarditis. There is a background of low-key protective mechanisms that typically keeps an every day, normal bacteraemia under control.[13] These protective mechanisms can be overcome by large numbers of bacteria. Bacteria may survive because of specific defects in the multiple, integrated systems that pertain to and affect specific organisms. Though general principles apply, there is no single mechanism of protection against all organisms.[14]

The functions of skin are not limited to maintenance of heat and body fluid while keeping the external environment out of the body. Skin participates in the general immunological response, its by-products are used throughout the body, it regulates temperature by giving off heat as well as conserving it, it absorbs substances, excretes substances, and it breathes. Indeed, the full function of the skin is unknown. It is the largest organ of the body, but is seldom looked upon as such except by those with a global concept of anatomy.

The skin is the barrier to the outside world and when it is gone the outside world enters unwanted. The goal of the burn team is to re-establish this barrier whether by substitution or by providing the circumstances that allow the skin to replace itself. During the interim, bacteria are at work trying to survive and in the process tend to become hostile to the host.

By far the most common site of infection in burn patients is the burn eschar. The reason patients become ill with the formation of eschar is not totally understood. Suffice it to say, there is a breakdown of systemic defence systems when the skin is lost, but it is not an all-or-nothing phenomenon. Patients become systemically septic, yet general defence systems may be intact when tested *in vitro*.[14] This is seen with whole blood, plasma, and white blood cell function. The typical burn patient begins to show signs and symptoms of being clinically infected between 5 to 7 days and remains susceptible until the wounds are closed.

Pick a number and wait

Teplitz defined burn wound sepsis as 100 000 organisms per gram of tissue.[15,16] This concept was central in the understanding of bacterial activity in the burn wound. At this concentration of bacteria, the local controlling effects of the wound are overpowered and the bacteria begin a systemic invasion. Teplitz worked with *P. aeruginosa* at a time when it was the major cause of infection in burn patients and a significant participant in their deaths.

The quantitative measurement of bacteria in the wound has become an integral part in the clinical care of patients. Variations and modifications to determine the presence of burn wound sepsis stem from Teplitz's original findings. Understanding of bacteria, however, has improved. Bacterial virulence has not been appreciated fully in the clinical environment. Though antibiotic resistance is encountered and identification of better drugs is sought for a patient, the bacteria do not always accommodate to the clinical situation. Where 1×10^5 may define burn wound sepsis for the original strain of *P. aeruginosa*, it is not necessarily the appropriate number for other bacteria.[14] There is evidence that, for virulent bacteria, the definition of burn wound sepsis may be a number less than 100 000, and for relatively avirulent bacteria a number greater than 100 000.[17]

As it has been shown that the number of bacteria in the wound is important, it is important that the test be properly done. The sensitivity of the bacteria to antibiotics is as important as the number present on the sample. When taking quantitative biopsies of the wound for bacterial counts, the area is infiltrated with a local anaesthetic that does not have a preservative, such as intracardiac lignocaine (lidocaine) hydrochloride. If the preservative is picked up with the specimen, it will be carried to the culture and inhibit growth of the bacteria. Recently, the rapid evaluation of slides of tissue has replaced the slower and older method of evaluating burn wound sepsis. If bacterial virulence is considered as part of the definition of burn wound sepsis, however, the presence of smaller numbers of bacteria capable of systemic spread makes for a more difficult evaluation of a pathology slide. Before the organisms can be seen by microscopy 100 000 bacteria may be present. The standard technique remains a quantitative count of bacteria in the wound. The relevance of the number is modified by the understanding of the bacterium's virulence.[15,16]

A journey begins with the first flip of a flagella

When bacteria spread systemically from the burn wound, they do so via the lymphatic channels which eventually lead to the central venous system. Bacteria subsequently gain access to the right heart and lungs, and typically are filtered from the blood by the lungs. If they escape the filtering, the bacteria go on to the left side of the heart and are ejected into the peripheral vascular system. Lastly, they reach the peripheral veins after passing through the capillaries. Blood cultures are typically taken from these peripheral veins. This long, Jasonian journey in part explains the lack of positive blood cultures in the face of clinical sepsis. There is local peri-arterial infiltration in tissue overwhelmed by the bacteria and this is a classic sign of *P. aeruginosa* pathology. These are local wound infections and do not originate from haematogenous spread.

Knowing that the skin and its eschar are the source of the majority of infections in burn patients leads to a significant effort directed toward control of that end. A burn wound is never sterile. The topical agents used are designed to keep the wound bacteria at a count below that of burn wound sepsis. Topical control is accomplished in two ways: mechanically and chemically. Soap and water washing is the most frequently used method of mechanically keeping a wound clean. The number of bacteria is kept low and systemic invasion is limited. The addition of a topical agent to a mechanical technique enhances wound control. Wet-to-dry dressings with Dakin's solution or a liquid antimicrobial such as silver nitrate are examples of both mechanical and chemical treatment of wounds.

Surgical control of bacteria consists of removing infected wound and eschar and covering the wound with skin or a skin substitute. The burn wound can be likened to an abscess, but instead of the abscess being inside the patient, the patient is inside the abscess needing to get out. Infected wounds are removed by tangential and full thickness excision. Tangential excision is the shaving of the wound down to bleeding, non-infected, viable tissue. Full thickness excision is removal of burned tissue down to the fascia, removing the dermal elements that would allow secondary closure of the wound.

The mortality of patients without inhalation injuries is improved by early wound excision.[18] The evolution of these techniques stems from work of those who saw the surgical process as a rapid means of closing limited size third degree burn wounds, without thought of their being infected.[19–24] Effective use of excision and topical agents to reduce bacterial counts on the wound has shifted the source of systemic sepsis from the wound toward the lungs and in some series has changed the cause of infection from bacterial to non-bacterial burn wound infections.[25]

The problems caused when a large burn wound is excised is the created open defect and how it can be closed. An open wound is susceptible to bacterial invasion. Autograft is the best solution; homograft is the second best solution; closure with substitutes, either topical medication or artificial skin substitutes, is the third best solution.

More than bargained for

The loss of skin has a total-body effect that goes beyond the local skin loss, as the immunological system is also affected. The size of the burn causing such a change varies with the age and the premorbid medical condition of the patient. In the establishment of an infection in a burn patient, there is an interplay of the host and the invading organism. Bacteria change and patients change. The ability of the host to combat infection will vary throughout the course of a disease; the ability of an organism to establish an infection will vary throughout a disease. A patient encountering a virulent organism early in the clinical course, when the majority of defence mechanisms are intact, will control a bacterial attack. A patient confronted with a relatively avirulent organism at a time when defence systems are exhausted or in disarray will be unable to ward off invasion. Timing of an infection helps explain why one patient will reject a virulent *Staphylococcus aureus* early in his clinical course, but will later succumb to a relatively avirulent *Candida albicans*. An organism responsible for the death of a patient, however, is not avirulent to that patient.

Pneumonia is frequently associated with inhalation injuries and is expected in patients that require prolonged intubation. Urinary tract infections are associated with Foley catheters. Intravenous line sites have a high frequency of infection,[26] and lines left in place for more than 72 hours in burn patients have a much higher incidence of infection. In general, tubes stuck into burn patients cause problems.

Indwelling tubes block the normal drainage of the channels they occupy. Endotracheal tubes fill the nasal passage, block sinus drainage, and lead to sinusitis and abscesses that cause occult fevers and sepsis. After an endotracheal tube is removed it is difficult to identify the source of sepsis weeks after respiratory support is no longer needed. Foley catheters can block the seminal vesicles and secretory ducts and can lead to epididymitis.

A special problem

Suppurative phlebitis is a complication of contaminated veins resulting in a vein filled with a column of pus that systemically seeds bacteria.[27] Such veins produce occult fevers days to weeks before the source is identified. Historically, the initiating intravenous line has been removed several weeks before the symptoms begin. Early diagnosis only occurs because of a high index of suspicion. The vein must be removed from its bed. Anything less is a compromise. The removed infected vein is followed up and into its major venous tributary. The peripheral veins are the most frequently involved. Attempting to make a diagnosis by aspiration with a needle stick is non-productive. The confirming diagnosis is made by noting a vessel the diameter of an adult's thumb that is surrounded by hot and inflamed tissue. The vein bed is left open and treated as an infected wound with wet-to-dry antimicrobial dressing and delayed closure. Occasionally, a skin graft is required to close the defect.

Central venous lines and Swan–Ganz catheters remain the paradox in the care of these patients. They are necessary for making decisions, but they are the frequent source of infection and other causes of complications in burn and trauma patients.[28] All invasive foreign materials are potential sites and sources for infection. They must be placed with forethought and removed as soon as they are no longer needed or informative.

What is it and how much is it going to cost?

The clinical diagnosis of infection and identification of the causative organism in burn patients can be difficult. Diagnosis of an infected burn patient is a qualitative and quantitative process. Frequently, treatment is directed by clinical signs and cues. This is not the quantitative information on which one would like to base decisions, but it is all too often the only information upon which to act. Glycosuria is an example of one of the more important clinical findings. Glycosuria in a patient known to have no previous evidence of diabetes is septic until proven otherwise. Antibiotics, not insulin, are the therapy of choice. Until sepsis is under control, the glucose metabolism will not be under control.

High fevers of 40 °C can be of value in making clinical decisions in burn patients. Fevers of 38.5 to 39.5 °C are not considered to be pathological but due to an increased metabolic rate. A practical problem is deciding when to take cultures from patients who have undulating fever curves. A thorough work-up includes cultures of the blood, urine, sputum, and the wound. It is both expensive and time consuming. There is no answer to the question of 'how many is enough?' The clinical decision is based on the situation at hand, recognizing that sepsis is the number one killer of burn patients. No one should be called to task for being conservative and taking cultures.

Mental disorientation and ileus are subtle signs and symptoms of sepsis. Either one by itself is inconclusive, but together they add to a definitive diagnosis.

Haematological changes with sepsis include a rise in the white blood cell count (WBC) and fall in platelet count. The WBC count is an excellent indicator for patients who have the ability to respond to infection with a leucocytosis. Burn patients, however, will exhaust their white cells and, when long into the clinical course, may not be able to mount a response. The elderly are particularly prone to have a septic disaster in progress, yet have a normal WBC count. If elevated, a count is of value; if normal, the value is to be viewed with suspicion. With sepsis secondary to gram negative organisms, the platelet count will be low. This can be an early indication of uncontrolled infection.

Cultures defining sepsis are often inconclusive, but patients can be physiologically evaluated by a Swan–Ganz catheter placed in the pulmonary artery for haemodynamic measurements. Typically a high cardiac output and a low peripheral vascular resistance confirms sepsis. The diagnosis is strengthened by an associated narrow arterial–venous oxygen difference (CaO_2–CvO_2) and is confirmed by an increased fluid requirement to maintain urinary output and blood pressure. In the face of such findings and no positive cultures, it is justifiable to treat with systemic antibiotics, choosing broad coverage for gram negative and gram positive bacteria. It is not the custom to give systemic medication to treat fungal infections until there are positive cultures because the available drugs are potentially toxic. Oral antifungal medication, however, is given to patients with large burns to inhibit fungal overgrowth in the GI tract.

Respiratory failure is defined both quantitatively and qualitatively. It is easier to recognize quantitative changes because numbers define cut-off points which facilitate decision-making. Arterial blood gases with:

$PaO_2 < 7.0$ kPa with an FiO_2 0.4–0.6 with oxygen supplementation and
$PaCO_2 > 7.0$ kPa (non-alkalotic compensation) require aggressive support.

There are, however, qualitative indications of respiratory failure associated with sepsis. Obstruction of the airway, atelectasis or lobar collapse, copious tracheobronchial secretions, and excessive work of breathing are a few indicators. The qualitative features can be distilled to a function of looking at the respiratory effort of the patient; if you get tired watching the patient breathe, respiratory support is needed.

Name, rank, and serial number

A positive wound culture is the *sine qua non* of defining sepsis in burn patients. Topical antimicrobial and surgical debridement are designed to reduce the number of bacteria on the wound; by keeping the number of bacteria low, a contaminated wound does not become an infected wound. Chemical agents directly interfere in bacterial metabolism. Surgical debridement mechanically removes bacteria and burn wound eschar.

Any positive culture is considered separately and with the clinical condition taken into account. *Staphylococcus epidermidis* is a clinical pathogen for burn patients. Controlling it can be difficult because its presence is associated with a compromised immunological system. *Staphylococcus aureus* is a frequent resident in burn wards, often resistant to methicillin, and thought to be a hospital acquired infection. Effective medications are limited and may be toxic to the patient. Though *S. aureus* is a present problem, it is not a new one. There is a cycle whereby organisms appear, disappear, and re-appear in the burn wards. The phenomenon is a consequence of changing antibiotics and the prolonged survival of patients with large wounds. Not only are 'old' bacteria returning to the burn wards, organisms that were never seen before are causing clinical problems such as HIV, *S. epidermidis* and *Acinetabacter*.

A non-bacterial organism which infects debilitated burn victims is the *Candida* species. Its presence is an ominous sign for a burn victim and is indicative of severe immunological compromise. Candida may be heralded by *S. epidermis* infection in the wounds or in blood. Once *Candida* is cultured from three sources, systemic treatment must be instigated. But treatment is begun with less than three positive culture sites when the patient has clinical signs of sepsis.

The treatment of *Candida* can be as menacing as the finding of the organism. To date, the most effective medication is amphotericin-B, but the side effects of hypersensitivity and renal failure can be as grave as the organism against which it is being given. A new medication, yet to be tried by time, is fluconazole. It can be given orally or intravenously, the oral being declared as effective as the intravenous form.

Herpes is a viral infection seen particularly, but not exclusively, in children. It has a dermatome distribution in its classic form. Cyclosporin is given for treatment. Typically the organism is not responsible for major complications or death in patients unless it is associated with an overwhelming sepsis. In such cases its effects are sublimated by the overwhelming complications of the major infecting organisms.[29,30]

Topical antimicrobials

Topical agents are used on open wounds to reduce the number of bacteria present; they do not sterilize the wound. Silver sulphadiazine is presently the most popular choice. It is water soluble and does not cause pain on application. It is associated with a leucopaenia early in the course of use, but the condition is reversed when the topical is stopped temporarily.[31,32] It seems that *Staphylococcus aureus* emerges through silver sulphadiazine. This phenomenon is anticipated with the intent of changing the medication if necessary. Mafenide is excellent for small injuries where penetration of the drug is desirable, such as a burned ear with relatively avascular cartilage. It is painful on the wound and the need for pain medication must be anticipated. It is a carbonic anhydrase inhibitor and is not placed on large surface defects, as metabolic acidosis will occur.

Additional topical agents with antimicrobial properties are povidone iodine, Dakin's solution (chloramine-T is the present-day substitute), silver nitrate, and other parochial substances. Povidone iodine is associated with iodine absorption from large burn wounds and is painful on application.[33,34] Chloramine-T now substitutes for the original Dakin's solution (sodium hypochlorite). It was used during World Ward I by Carrel in the treatment of wounds.[35] Carrel's principle of wound debridement is as true today as when it was controversially proposed.

Silver nitrate as 0.5% solution remains an effective topical agent against burn wound bacteria. It readily precipitates as silver chloride when in contact with the sodium of wounds and is rendered ineffective. The silver solution is best warmed so as not to cool the patient. It requires frequent application and this will affect patterns of nursing care. Additionally it stains the patient, the equipment, and the hospital. In spite of all these faults, it remains a solution against which bacteria have not developed a resistance. There has been renewed interest because of recent work with silver using a weak direct electric current across a *Pseudomonas aeruginosa* infected wound which resulted in a reduced incidence of fatal burn wound sepsis.[36]

Systemic antimicrobials

Systemic antibiotics are given for two general conditions, for prophylaxis and loss of local control from specific organisms leading to systemic invasion. Treatment is most effective when the antibiotic chosen is effective against identified pathogens.[37] Prophylactic antibiotics are not given indiscriminately to all burn patients. The experience has been that virulent, resistant organisms will emerge and sweep through burn care facilities, killing patients with ever more ease. There is a documented increase in donor site infections when perioperative antibiotics are not given.[38]

Sub-eschar injection is a combination of systemic and topical antibiotic use.[39] Historically, this was used before excision of burn eschar was widely practised. The practice is effective because it changes the pH of the wound, allowing inherent protective systems to function properly in a physiologically normal environment.[40]

Mechanical care

Soap and water washing is the simplest of the mechanical techniques as it reduces the number of bacteria on the wound. Wet-to-dry dressings is a similar mechanical process. Saline, which has no antimicrobial properties, or agents such as povidone iodine or Dakin's solution which do have antimicrobial properties, are liquids used in the technique.

The ultimate mechanical wound care for the surgeon is an operation. There are two techniques in his armamentarium, excision and grafting. Excision can be either tangential or full thickness. Tangential excision is the shaving of the eschar from the burn wound until down to bleeding, viable tissue. The danger is loss of too much blood. As a consequence tourniquets have been proposed, but they do not affect the final outcome in blood loss.[41] The blood loss from excision is estimated at 200 millilitres per percent surface area and will limit the area of wound that can be excised during one operation.[42] Though there are reports of giving several blood volume replacements and operating for up to seven hours during a single excision, most institutions and patients are not subjected to such treatment.[43] The danger of such techniques is that the number of significant infections increases directly proportional to the number of red cell transfusions.[44]

Full thickness excision is done with a hot knife and at a deeper level of the skin, between the subdermal fat and fascia. At this depth, the blood vessels do not have as much arborization as at the more superficial level. Control of bleeding is greater than with tangential excision, therefore larger areas of the body can be excised during a single operation.

Healthy tissue left exposed by tangential and full thickness excision has to be protected from becoming infected. Surgeons are taught not to place grafts on blood filled recipient beds, yet with freshly excised burn wounds, autograft has a haemostatic effect. As a consequence, freshly excised wounds are immediately autografted if skin is available. This protects the wound from resulting infection and obviates further operations when the grafting is successful. A grossly contaminated wound with surrounding cellulitis with its related phenomena of rubor, calor, dolor, tumor, and functio laesa must not be grafted immediately, even if autograft is available.

If autograft is not available to protect the excised defect, homograft is a substitute. Although the donor has given an ultimate gift, homograft must not be looked at as being indispensable. If there is infection of the wound after its placement, the homograft is removed and the wound covered with fresh homograft or by a topical antimicrobial.

Prophylaxis

Polyvalent and divalent vaccines against specific organisms have been developed, but they have not been clinically practical.[45,46] Painting wounds with an immunomodulator prior to inoculation can reduce the incidence of wound infection.[47] But the clinical conundrum is, how are burn victims prepared for an unknown disease? Because burn trauma diminishes the immunological response, vaccines given to critically burned patients are not readily utilized to actively produce antibodies. Most clinical work has been attempted with vaccines against *Pseudomonas aeruginosa* but this has not proved successful.

Special problems of the day: fighting in the dark

Increasing numbers of patients on the burn ward will have human immunodeficiency virus (HIV). They represent medical, ethical, and legal problems to the treating team. In the United States, it is not presently allowable to test for the disease unless the patient gives fully informed consent. Therefore, alternative methods are used to confirm a suspected infection. Patients with acquired immunodeficiency disease (AIDS) have the findings of opportunistic infections and associated cancers such as Kaposi's sarcoma or non-Hodgkin's lymphoma. *Pneumocystis carinii* pneumonia and toxoplasmosis are commonly also associated with AIDS.

Between the extremes of plasma positive for HIV and terminal AIDS is the condition of AIDS-related Complex (ARC). This is associated with persistent lymphadenopathy, wasting, fevers, oral thrush (candidiasis), and other symptomatic findings. The diagnosis of ARC is made indirectly by culturing the opportunistic organisms or identifying them in a typical anatomical location, such as oesophageal candidiasis by way of endoscopy. Suspicion of the disease occurs when a burn patient consumes excessive amounts of food, yet does not gain weight or heal their wounds.

Afterthoughts

Bacteria are the oldest known living cells and as such are worthy of admiration and awe. To think they can be out-thought and out-done is to be naive. Bacteria are adaptive, genetically smart. They have been able to endure and avoid annihilation. Watch carefully and quietly and a great deal can be learnt from them about survival.

References

1 Stratta RJ, Warden GD, Ninnemann JL, Saffle JR. Immunologic parameters in burned patients: effects of therapeutic interventions. *J Trauma* 1986; **26**:7–17.

2 Forsberg CM and Bullen JJ: The effect of passage and iron on the virulence of *Pseudomonas aeruginosa. J Clin Path* 1972; **25**:65–8.
3 Bullen JJ, Ward CG, Wallis SN. Virulence and the role of iron in *Pseudomonas aeruginosa* infection. *Infect Immun* 1974; **10**:443–50.
4 Forsberg CM. The study on the mechanisms of resistance to *Pseudomonas aeruginosa* infections. PhD Thesis, Council for National Academic Awards, National Institute for Medical Research, London, August,1972.
5 Kominos SD, Copeland CE, Grosiak B, Postic B. Introduction of *Pseudomonas aeruginosa* into a hospital via vegetables. *Appl Microbiol* 1972; **24**:567–70.
6 Kominos SD, Copeland CE, Grosiak B. Mode of transmission of *Pseudomonas aeruginosa* in a burn unit and an intensive care unit in a general hospital. *Appl Microbiol* 1972; **23**:309–12.
7 Wright MP, Taddonio TE, Prasad JK, Thomson PD. The microbiology and cleaning of thermoplastic splints in burn care. *J Burn Care & Rehabil* 1989; **10**:79–83.
8 Berg RD, Garlington AW. Translocation of certain indigenous bacteria from the gastrointestinal tract to the mesenteric lymph nodes and other organs in a gnotobiotic mouse animal. *Infect Immun* 1979; **23**:402–11.
9 Border JR, Hassett J, LaDuca J *et al.* Gut origin septic states in blunt multiple trauma (ISS = 40) in the ICU. *Ann Surg* 1987; **206**:427–46.
10 Deitch EA, Ma L, Ma J-W, Berg RD. Lethal burn-induced bacterial translocation: role of genetic resistance. *J Trauma* 1989; **29**:1480–7.
11 Alverdy JC, Aoys E, Moss GS. Total parenteral nutrition promotes bacterial translocation from the gut. *Surgery* 1988; **104**:185–90.
12 Alexander JW, Boyce ST, Babcock LG, Peck MD *et al.* The process of microbial translocation. *Ann Surg* 1990; **212**:496–512.
13 Ward CG, Hammond, JS, Bullen JJ. Effect of iron on antibacterial function of human polymorphs and plasma. *Infect Immun* 1986; **51**:723–30.
14 Ward CG, Spalding PB, Marcial E, Bullen JJ. The bactericidal power of blood and plasma of patients with burns. *J Burn Care & Rehabil* 1991; **12**:120–6.15 Teplitz C, Davis D, Mason AD Jr, Moncrief JA.
15 Teplitz C, Davis D, Mason AD Jr, Moncrief JA. *Pseudomonas* burn wound sepsis. I. Pathogenesis of experimental *Pseudomonas* burn wound sepsis. *J Surg Res* 1964; **4**:200.
16 Teplitz C, Davis D, Walker HL, Raulston GL, Mason AD, Moncrief JA. *Pseudomonas* burn wound sepsis. II. *J Surg Res* 1964; **4**:217.
17 Ward CG, Bullen JJ, Spalding PB. Bacterial virulence and host selection: bacteria 'select' patients to infect. *J Burn Care & Rehabil* 1991; **12**:127–31.
18 Herndon DN, Barrow RE, Rutan RL, DesaiMH, Abston S. Comparison of conservative versus early excision. Therapies in severely burned patients. *Ann Surg* 1989; **209**:547–52.
19 Cope O, Laugohr J, Moore FD, Webster R. Expeditious care of full thickness burn wounds by surgical excision and grafting. *Ann Surg* 1947; **125**:1.
20 Haynes BW Jr: Early excision and grafting in third degree burns. *Trans South Surg Assoc* 1969; **80**:103.
21 Hendren WH, Constable JD, Zawacki BE. Early partial excision of major burns in children. *J Pediat Surg* 1968; **3**:445.
22 Hermans RP. Primary excision of full-thickness burns up to 40 percent of body surface followed immediately by micro- or meshgrafts. In: *Basic*

Problems in Burns. Vrabec R, Konickova Z, Moserova J (eds). Springer Verlag, Berlin, 1975.

23 Janzekovic Z. A new concept in grafting of burns. *J Trauma* 1970; **10**:1103.

24 Janzekovic Z. The burn wound from the surgical point of view. *J Trauma* 1975; **15**:42–62.

25 McManus WF, Mason AD Jr, Pruitt BA Jr. Excision of the burn wound in patients with large burns. *Arch Surg* 1989; **124**:718–729.

26 Franceschi D, Gerding RL, Phillips G, Fratianne RB. Risk factors associated with intravascular catheter infections in burned patients: a prospective, randomized study. *J Trauma* 1989; **29**:811–16.

27 Hammond, JS, Varas R, Ward CG. Suppurative thrombophlebitis: a new look at a continuing problem. *South Med J* 1988; **81**:969–71.

28 Ferguson M, Max MH, Marshall W. Emergency department infraclavicular subclavian vein catheterization in patients with multiple injuries and burns. *South Med J* 1988; **81**:433–5.

29 Kagan JR, Naraqi S, Matsuda T, Jonasson OM. Herpes simplex virus and cytomegalovirus infections in burn patients. *J Trauma* 1985; **25**:40–5.

30 Pruitt BA Jr. The diagnosis and treatment of infection in the burn patient. *J Burns* 1984; **11**:79–91.

31 Chan CK, Jarrett F, Moylan JA. Acute leucopenia as an allergic reaction to silver sulfadiazine in burn patients. *J Trauma* 1976; **16**:395–6.

32 Fuller FW, Engler PE. Leucopenia in non-septic burn patients receiving topical 1% silver sulfadiazine cream therapy: a survey. *J Burn Care & Rehabil* 1988; **9**:606–9.

33 Ward, CG. Hypernatremia and hyperosmolarity associated with topical povidone–iodine therapy. Abstract presented at the Tenth Annual Meeting of the American Burn Association, Birmingham, Alabama, 1978.

34 Matsuda T, Kharwadkar R, Hanumadass M, Appavu S, Krauss T. The serum iodine level in burn patients treated with topical povidone–iodine. Abstract; presented at Ninth Annual Meeting of the American Burn Association, Anaheim, California, 1977.

35 Malinin TI. *Surgery and Life, the Extraordinary Career of Alexis Carrel.* pp 65–81. Harcourt Brace Jovanovich, New York, NY, 1979.

36 Chu CS, McManus AT, Pruitt BA Jr, Mason AD Jr. Therapeutic effects of silver nylon dressings with weak direct current on *Pseudomonas aeruginosa*-infected burn wounds. *J Trauma* 1988; **28**:1488–92.

37 Dacso CC, Luterman A, Curreri PW. Systemic antibiotic treatment in burned patients. *Surg Clin N Am* 1987; **67**:57–68.

38 Griswold JA, Grube BJ, Engrave LH, Marvin JA, Heimbach DM. Determinants of donor site infections in small burn grafts. *J Burn Care & Rehabil* 1989; **10**:531–5.

39 Baxter CR, Curreri PW, Marvin JA. The control of burn wound sepsis by the use of quantitative bacteriologic studies and subeschar clysis with antibiotics. *Surg Clin N Am* 1973; **53**:1509–18.

40 Baxter CR. 'Right, but for the wrong reason!' *J Burn Care & Rehabil* 1988; **9**:457.

41 Thompson P, Herndon DN, Abston S, Rutan T. Effect of early excision on patients with major thermal injury. *J Trauma* 1987; **27**:205–7.

42 Moran KT, O'Reilly TJ, Furman W, Munster AM. A new algorithm for calculation of blood loss in excisional burn surgery. *Am Surg* 1988; **54**:207–8.

43 Chicarilli ZN, Cuono CB, Heinrich JJ, Fichandler BC, Barese S. Selective aggressive burn excision for high mortality subgroups. *J Trauma* 1986; **26**:18–25.

44 Graves TA, Cioffi WG, Mason AD Jr, Pruitt BA Jr. Relationship of transfusion and infection in a burn population. *J Trauma* 1989; **29**:948–52.

45 Holder IA, Naglich JC. Experimental studies of the pathogenesis of infections due to *Pseudomonas aeruginosa*: immunization using divalent flagella preparations. *J Trauma* 1986; **26**:118–22.

46 Jones RJ, Roe E, Gupta J. Controlled trials of a polyvalent *Pseudomonas* vaccine in burns. *Lancet* 1979; **i**:977–84.

47 Hershman MJ, Sonnenfeld G, Logan WA, Pietsch JD, Wellhausen SR, Polk HC Jr. Effect of interferongamma treatment on the course of a burn wound infection. *J Interferon Res* 1988; **8**:367–73.

10

Anaesthesia for the burned patient

L.T.A. RYLAH, S.M. UNDERWOOD

Introduction

The burned patient, when considered for an anaesthetic assessment, must be regarded as suffering from a most severe form of trauma and all the principles of assessment, resuscitation and treatment associated with multiple trauma must be followed. There may be other injuries sustained at the time of the burn, including inhalation, which will have to be dealt with during the resuscitation period. The benefits of anaesthesia and surgery must always outweigh the risks when all relevant information is taken into account.

There are three periods during which the burned patient may undergo anaesthesia for a surgical procedure. These are:

Immediate – From the time of the injury until cardiovascular stability has been established
Early – After resuscitation, 2–7 days post-burn
Late – More than 2 weeks post-burn.

There are major similarities between all three periods but each has different facets which may affect the type of anaesthesia chosen for the varied procedures that need to be carried out.

The immediate period

This period may last up to 48 hours from the time of the burn. There are two indications for operating at this time and they are at either end of the severity spectrum. If a major burn has been sustained, anaesthesia must only be contemplated if other trauma has caused a life-threatening situation which can only be remedied by surgery. If possible, resuscitation and stabilization must be completed prior to surgery. The second reason for operating would be to debride a small wound in a fit, healthy patient with minimal physiological disturbance. First, the major burn and associated trauma or life-threatening problems.

The pre-operative assessment

The type of trauma suffered by the patient must be accurately assessed. Blood loss from open wounds and fractures must be replaced in addition to the resuscitation fluids. Respiratory function may have been put in jeopardy by the inhalation of hot, toxic fumes or gases.[1] If a patient is suspected of having sustained an inhalational injury intubation is mandatory at the earliest possible time. This will protect the airway and allow higher concentrations of inspired oxygen to be delivered if necessary. Mechanical ventilation will allow the blood gas chemistry to be optimized. It must be remembered that a tracheal tube can easily be removed after the resuscitation period, if it is not required, but that it may prove impossible to place one later in the resuscitation phase when tissue oedema has appeared. This may, of course, lead to the demise of the patient due to obstruction of the airway. Suxamethonium is not contra-indicated during the first 24 hours and can be used to facilitate tracheal intubation.

A full medical history must be obtained, preferably before anaesthesia is commenced. In addition, these questions need to be answered:

At what time did the incident occur?
What is the age, weight, and percentage burn?
Where did it happen – enclosed or open space?
What type of heat exposure occurred?
Was there any burning material, i.e. wood, plastic, rubber?
If an electrical burn, what voltage was discharged?
Any complicating factors, i.e. associated trauma, cardiac arrest, arrhythmias?
Is there any airway problem or evidence of inhalation?
What resuscitation fluid has been given, and is there a deficit?
Is the procedure really necessary, and is there time to stabilize the patient?

The patient must undergo a quick but full examination to verify the information already obtained. At this time, the available venous access can be ascertained and improved if necessary.

Premedication

The patient is likely to be very ill or even moribund, making pre-medication unnecessary. If the surgery is urgent, there will be no time for premedication. Any medication given, however, must be via the intra-venous route as intramuscular injections will have an erratic absorption and be unreliable.[2]

Induction

As in trauma surgery, it is preferable to have stabilized the patient with a systolic blood pressure above 100 mmHg and a pulse rate below 100 beats per minute before commencing anaesthesia. However, this is often impossible. The agent of choice may be ketamine as it has positive inotropic and chronotropic effects, or etomidate which has less cardiac destabilizing action than methohexitone, thiopentone and propofol. A rapid sequence induction can be facilitated with suxamethonium, but only in the first 24 hours after the burn. An intubating dose of competitive muscle relaxant may be used if there are no apparent or potential airway problems.

Maintenance

All urgent burn trauma patients must be intubated and mechanically ventilated perioperatively. If the patient is moribund, oxygen alone is given to maintain adequate oxygen delivery. If the situation allows, nitrous oxide may be used and an inhalational agent may be contemplated to maintain anaesthesia. If adjunct gases are not used, enough opiate or opioid must be given to obtain some form of analgesia and amnesia. Fentanyl is probably the agent of choice[3] in a moderate to high dose, 10–20 μg/kg. The respiratory depressant effect of such a large dose need not hinder this technique as these patients will invariably need postoperative intensive care facilities and mechanical ventilation. If there is massive blood loss both the analgesic agent and muscle relaxant must be given in large doses and more frequently than usual as they are also lost. Muscle relaxants are a personal choice but for trauma patients pancuronium is most often selected. Atracurium[4] and vecuronium[5] may be used and have some advantages in certain circumstances. Tubocurare is generally contra-indicated now that more acceptable drugs are available.

Special requirements

There are special requirements which must be met for burns anaesthesia. Although some are common to all three periods, some are of greater importance than others in each period.

Personnel

There must be two anaesthetists present for any major trauma or burn patient. They must be experienced and of the highest calibre available.

Intravenous access

This must be secured before the commencement of anaesthesia. There must be two large-bore cannulae *in situ* for acute burn trauma cases as the need for rapid transfusion must be anticipated. If a clear site is present, and time is available, it is wise to insert a pulmonary artery catheter introducer to obtain central venous access and to allow replacement of large volumes of fluid in a short space of time. Then if it becomes necessary, a pulmonary artery catheter can be easily inserted to monitor the resuscitation, replacement of blood, cardiac output and other derived cardiovascular parameters.

Blood/fluid replacement

It is advisable to start blood replacement immediately. Any pre-operative loss must be replaced and the replacement of anticipated loss can be started in advance. The worst scenario is that of being unable to keep up with blood loss and trying to catch up when already behind. Even with the best intentions and preparations, this will happen occasionally.

Temperature maintenance

Heat loss is a major problem with any form of trauma.[6] The incident may have occurred in a cold environment, the victim may have been dowsed in cold water or may have lost heat through inadequate insulation on transfer. It is imperative that the patient be kept at a normal temperature, thus every effort must be made to avoid heat loss. The operating theatre must be warmed, preparation fluids warmed to body temperature, all intravenous fluids passed through a blood warming device, inhaled gases humidified and warmed[7] and areas of the body not being operated upon must be kept covered at all times. Warming blankets[8] and overhead infrared heaters may be used but have their limitations. Core and peripheral temperatures must be monitored and kept as near normal as possible.

Monitoring

The level of monitoring must justify the severity of the injury. Basic monitoring of pulse rate, electrocardiography, skin and core temperatures and non-invasive blood pressure is mandatory in all cases. Non-invasive techniques may be impossible if the burn affects all limbs although it may be possible to rotate the cuff to limbs not being operated on. Invasive arterial blood pressure monitoring, if available, must be used in severe burns as wave form and beat to beat variation greatly aid the management of fluid replacement. A pulmonary artery catheter may be necessary if there is doubt about the adequacy of fluid replacement. Ventilatory monitoring of inspired oxygen concentration, end tidal carbon dioxide levels, ventilator pressures and pulse oximetry are advised. Serial blood gas analyses are useful when an inhalation injury has occurred, and where a pulmonary artery catheter is in place the calculation of an oxygen extraction ratio is extremely helpful.

Urine output

This must be monitored throughout the immediate period and will be an indicator of adequate resuscitation.[9] It must be kept greater than 0.5 ml/kg/h without the use of diuretics. Insertion of a urinary catheter is mandatory.

Haemostasis

A consumptive coagulopathy will occur at the same time as a dilution effect.[10] This is adequately treated with large volumes of fresh frozen plasma. In practice it would be wasteful to use such a resource whilst the patient is undergoing surgery. It is therefore advised that the blood loss be replaced until surgical haemostasis is secured, then the clotting defect is corrected with fresh frozen plasma. Any replacement during surgery would be ineffective and wasteful.

Postoperative care

This must be on the Critical Care Unit. Mechanical ventilation is advised in the postoperative period as oxygen delivery can be monitored adequately and the patient can have adequate analgesia and sedation without compromising the airway or respiratory function. Postoperative cardiovascular stabilization may involve invasive monitoring techniques, including pulmonary artery catheterization, accompanied by cardiovascular manipulation using both fluid replacement and inotropes. If these procedures are performed, it is unlikely that the awake, anxious patient will co-operate and therefore sedation is indicated.

Physiological parameters

These must be optimized. A dynamic approach must be taken to blood and fluid replacement as well as oxygen supply and demand. Monitoring of blood gases, electrolytes, haemoglobin, haematocrit and clotting parameters must be frequent and remedial action taken as early as possible.

The small burn

A patient may be received with a burn that has caused minimal physiological upset. Heat loss will be minimal, resuscitation good and there may be no pre-existing complicating factors. Debridement at this stage may present minimal anaesthetic risks and will convert a burn into a straightforward trauma case. Consequently, postoperative fluid management will not follow a resuscitation regime as long as intra-operative volume replacement has been adequate. This may lead to a saving in the use of resuscitation fluids,[11] particularly plasma. Blood loss is more excessive when operating early and this must be anticipated. The special requirements already described may be relevant but must be scaled down for a lesser injury. The anaesthetic technique will more closely resemble that used in the early, post-resuscitation period.

The early period

This would normally be the time when a burned patient commences surgical treatment. Resuscitation will have been successfully completed and the patient will be ready to undergo anaesthesia with decreased risk. Debridement of all burned tissue is performed as soon as is feasible.

Pre-operative assessment

The patient will have been under close observation for over 48 hours. The information obtained on admission will be important, but additional questions will need to be answered and these answers taken into account when planning the anaesthetic technique. The response of the patient to resuscitation must be noted: adequate renal function is a good indicator of this. The airway needs to be examined as swelling or inhalation may change the course of treatment. Venous access must be examined and additional or replacement cannulae inserted and secured if necessary. A standard check on haemoglobin, haematocrit, urea, electrolytes and clotting function must be performed. Finally, communication with the surgeon is mandatory; the extent of the surgery must be ascertained, the likely blood loss estimated (he will usually underestimate!) and the positioning or anticipated moving of the patient during the operation must be considered. A picture can then be built up of the problems that may occur during the course of anaesthesia. If the patient is mechanically ventilated, the anaesthesia can be considered to be an extension of the sedative/analgesic regime in progress.

Premedication

The main aim of the burn anaesthetist is to secure patient recovery with minimal hangover in the shortest possible time. These patients are already on analgesia and hopefully have come to terms with their injury. For this reason no premedicant drugs are given unless there is a specific request or indication. Normal analgesia, however, must not be withheld prior to surgery.

Induction

If the vascular access obtained for resuscitation is no longer present at least one, if not two, large-bore cannulae must be positioned. Two cannulae are essential for a major excision and grafting procedure. The patient should be taken to the operating room on the ward bed and induction performed on the bed if local procedures allow. Thus the patient can be transferred after induction of anaesthesia, avoiding un-necessary pain on movement. A large dose of the chosen analgesic agent must be given prior to induction. Fentanyl is an excellent drug for this purpose and, given in a dose of 10–15 μg/kg, will supply good operative analgesia which may carry into the postoperative period, depending on the duration and extent of the surgical procedure. Droperidol may be given at this time in an anti-emetic dose range but is not usually necessary. As long as the cardiovascular system is stable, propofol is the induction agent of choice[12] as it allows a short recovery without hangover.[13] Atracurium is the relaxant to use for maintenance and given at 0.6 mg/kg provides adequate relaxation for intubation. Suxamethonium is contra-indicated as a sudden rise in plasma potassium will occur and may cause cardiac arrest and death. Vecuronium may be used but, after long operations, when a large dose has been administered, accumulation of drug may make relaxation difficult to reverse. Before the introduction of atracurium and vecuronium mixtures of curare and pancuronium (cura-lon) were used to offset the cumulative effects of each in an attempt to make reversal easier.[14] This mixture should be considered where the newer relaxants are not available.

Intubation

If facial burns are present care must be taken when siting the tracheal tube. The position and type of tube used must be discussed with the surgeon as surgery to the face may be contemplated. Securing the tube may present a problem as a tie may have to be very loose or may not be feasible. A nasotracheal tube may be required and will be more secure than an oral tube if untied.

Maintenance

Analgesia is very important as these patients will undergo many surgical procedures. If excess pain is experienced each procedure will be feared. Thus the patient must feel confident that pain will be kept to a minimum. Enough analgesia must be given for this purpose and it is better to mechanically ventilate a patient for a few hours postoperatively than to reverse the effects of a relative excess of analgesic agent. However, due to the large requirements of analgesic and severe pain experienced, respir-atory depression is very rare. Increments of fentanyl, to supplement the dose given prior to induction, will provide good analgesia. If morphine or papaveretum have been used as analgesia prior to surgery, it may be sensible to continue them perioperatively and into the postoperative period. In the UK, phenoperidine is available and its longer action may be advantageous. However, it must be borne in mind that phenoperidine has a stronger depressant effect on respiration.

Isoflurane is the inhalational agent of choice for maintenance. It gives a fast recovery with little nausea. However, the other inhalational agents may also be used. As to date, no documented case of hepatitis following multiple halothane anaesthesia has been recorded in a burned patient[15,16] and, if not otherwise contra-indicated, halothane is one of the safest agents to use.

Nitrous oxide has been shown to cause suppression of bone marrow,[17] although this may be insignificant when compared with the impairment of erythropoiesis caused by the burn itself. Air and oxygen mixture is the carrier gas of choice both medically and environmentally. It is wise to aspirate the stomach via a nasogastric tube to withdraw any gases or inhalational agents that may have been introduced during hand ventilation prior to intubation. This will decrease the incidence of postoperative nausea and vomiting.

Upon termination of the surgical procedure, it is humane to transfer the patient from the operating table onto the ward bed before reversing the muscle relaxant and terminating the anaesthetic. If atracurium or vecuronium have been used, reversal is not usually a problem and, in practice, reversal agents are rarely necessary. Neostigmine, together with either atropine or glycopyrrolate, provide an acceptable reversal mixture. Pharyngeal suction must be performed and a Guedel-type airway inserted. Extubation must only be performed when the patient is adequately reversed and breathing spontaneously, as in any other branch of anaesthesia.

If the patient awakes in excessive pain, the analgesic of choice must be titrated intravenously by the anaesthetist as a matter of urgency.

Special requirements

These are mainly the same as those during the immediate phase, i.e. monitoring, temperature control, clotting function, intravenous access, fluid balance and blood replacement. After a large operation, the patient must be sedated and mechanically ventilated. This will allow the administration of adequate analgesia and provide a patient in whom cardiovascular manipulations can be carried out without the patient becoming unduly anxious.

Postoperative pyrexia is common but should settle between 24 and 36 hours. These pyrexias must be treated with suspicion and those persisting, or occurring after this time, must be investigated formally and treated adequately.

Any excision exceeding 20% total body surface area (TBSA) will result in a consumptive coagulopathy requiring treatment with fresh frozen plasma and possibly platelets. However, this must not be confused with surgical blood loss due to inadequate haemostasis. Excessive bleeding must be examined both visually and haematologically. Most burn units limit their excisions to 20% TBSA for each visit to theatre in order to reduce this problem. The amount of excision to be performed must be discussed between the surgeon and intensivist when planning the course of treatment.

Dressing changes

There is a period of time between major operations, in either the early or later phase of treatment, when burned patients may have to undergo painful, undignified or even embarrassing procedures. The removal of dressings in a bath surrounded by many nurses may be painful, and for most patients will result in some loss of dignity. Removal of dressings and other procedures may be performed more quickly and with less man-power if performed under general anaesthesia. Thus a technique has been developed for a patient to be anaesthetized without going to the operating room. Normal precautions must be observed; equipment for airway management, suction and oxygen must be to hand. Monitoring must, at least, consist of electrocardiography and pulse oximetry. A patent intravenous cannula must be in situ. Alfentanil, at approximately 10 mcg/kg, is given intravenously and, once its effect has been noted, induction is commenced using a sleep dose of propofol. The patient is allowed to breathe oxygen-enriched air after the insertion of a Guedel airway. Incremental propofol is given to maintain unconsciousness, care being taken not to cause apnoea. Some slight voluntary reflex movement by the patient is tolerated. If the procedure is short, not painful, or if other analgesics are in progress, alfentanil is omitted. The patient must be starved overnight and the procedure carried out as early as possible to minimize the starvation period. The patient is usually ready for breakfast within 30 minutes of the end of anaesthesia. This technique has proved especially useful in children, for the removal of skin staples and removal or change of dressings on both donor and graft sites. Once the dressings have been removed, the patient is allowed to awake as the pain experienced during application of new dressings is usually acceptable to all concerned.

The late period

Modern treatment of the burn usually entails early tangential excision. However, there may have been reasons to allow the wound to deslough.

These will probably have been concurrent medical or surgical problems, or difficult or unsuccessful resuscitation. There will come a time when an operative procedure is necessary and this then falls into the late phase. There may be significant peri-operative blood loss but it is usually less than during the early phase. Infection may have set in or be dormant and may lead to a disseminated intravascular coagulation for which control of the sepsis (wound debridement, antibiotics and fresh frozen plasma) will be the only course of treatment.

There is a second cohort of patients requiring an operation during this phase. For these patients, early excision and grafting will have gained skin cover but some then require more grafting, reconstructive surgery or 'tidying up' procedures. This phase, as intimated, will merge imperceptibly into the reconstructive phase when the techniques of anaesthesia border on those used for plastic surgery. The restoration of form and function may entail a course of surgery extending over a period of many years.

All the points made so far have to be addressed. Again, it is advisable to avoid suxamethonium since it may cause problems in patients long after skin coverage has been completed.[18,19] Skin grafts, especially recent ones, are fragile and susceptible to pressure and sheering forces. Positioning and handling of patients must be performed with great care. Grafts to the face and neck, as well as contractures, make airway management difficult and the likelihood of a difficult intubation must always be considered. A difficult intubation drill must be formulated and the relevant equipment available. An experienced surgeon must be in the room in the event that surgical intervention is necessary to secure the airway. Fluid balance, heat loss and monitoring have all been mentioned previously. The monitoring level must be justified by the scope and severity of the surgical procedure. It may be necessary to insert arterial lines and a pulmonary artery catheter but it must be stressed that these invasive techniques must be discontinued when the parameters they produce are no longer useful. They must not be left *in situ* just for convenience because they represent an increased risk of infection.

Problems associated with the reconstructive phase are beyond the scope of this chapter as they fall into the sphere of plastic anaesthetic techniques.

Summary

Anaesthesia for the burned patient is a specialized branch of anaesthesia somewhat akin to trauma anaesthesia. The major problems of burned patients are their fluid balance, blood loss and replacement, temperature control and analgesia. Monitoring may be a problem, even impossible, and experience is essential. Burned patients range in age from neonates to the elderly and will have all known medical problems with which the burn anaesthetist must be conversant. Finally, the treatment of burned patients is stressful to all staff and it is essential that the burn anaesthetist is part of the burn team in all aspects.

References

1 Achauer BM, Allyn PA, Furnas DW, Bartlett RH. Pulmonary complications of burns: the major threat to the burn patient. *Ann Surg* 1973; **177**:311–19.
2 Nancekievill D. Pain relief in emergencies. *Care Crit Ill* 1985; **1(4)**:222–4.
3 Watson CB, Norfleet EA. Anaesthesia for trauma. *Crit Care Clin* 1986; **2(4)**:717–46.
4 Hughes R. Atracurium – the first years. *Clin Anaesthesiol* 1985; **3(2)**:331–45.
5 Baird WLM, Savage DS. Vercuronium – the first years. *Clin Anaesthesiol* 1985; **3(2)**:347–60.
6 Luna GK, Maier RV, Pavin EG, Anardi D, Copass MK, Oreskovich MR. Incidence and effect of hypothermia in seriously injured patients. *J Trauma* 1987; **27**:1014–18.
7 Stone DR, Downs JB, Paul WL, Perkins HM. Adult body temperature and heated humidification of anaesthetic gases during general anaesthesia. *Anaesth and Analg* 1981; **60**:736–41.
8 Morris RH, Kumar A. The effect of warming blankets on maintenance of body temperature of the anesthetized, paralyzed patient. *Anesthesiology* 1972; **36**:408–11.
9 Settle JAD. Urine output following severe burns. *Burns* 1974; **1**:23–42.
10 Stoetling RK, Miller RD. Fluid and blood therapy, 256–57. In: *Basics of Anesthesia*, Churchill Livingstone, New York, NY. 1989.
11 Frame JD, Taweepoke P, Moimen N, Rylah L. Immediate facial flap reconstruction of joint use of Biobrane in the burned limb. *Burns* 1990; **16**:381–4.
12 Fahy LT, van Mourik GA, Utting JE. A comparison of the induction characteristics of thiopentone and propofol (2,6-di-isopropyl phenol). *Anaesthesia* 1985; **40**:939–40.
13 Grant IS, Mackenzie N. Recovery following propofol ('Diprivan') anaesthesia – a review of 3 different anaesthetic techniques. *Postgrad Med J* 1985; **61(3)**:133–7.
14 Satwicz PR, Martyn JAJ, Szyfelbein SK, Firestone S. Potentiation of neuromuscular blockade using a combination of pancuronium and dimethylcurarine. *Br J Anaesth* 1984; **56**:479–84.
15 Gronert GA, Schaneer PJ, Gunther RC. Multiple halothane anesthesia in the burn patient. *J Am Med Assn* 1968; **205**:878–9.
16 Martyn JAJ. Clinical pharmacology and therapeutics in burns, 190. In: *Acute Management of Burn Trauma*. Martyn JAJ (ed). WB Saunders, Philadelphia, PA, 1990.

17 Skacel PO, Hewlett AM, Lewis JD, Lumb M, Nunn JF, Chanarin I. Studies on the haemopoietic toxicity of nitrous oxide in man. *Br J Haematol* 1983; **53**:189–200.

18 Gronert GA, Theye RA. Pathophysiology of hyperkalaemia induced by succinylcholine. *Anesthesiology* 1975; **43**:89–99.

19 Martyn JAJ. Clinical pharmacology and therapeutics in burns, 195. In: *Acute Management of Burn Trauma*. Martyn JAJ (ed). WB Saunders, Philadelphia, PA, 1990.

11

Surgical management

G.D. WARDEN

Introduction

Historical perspective

Since the days of Hippocrates, traumatic wound management has been based on the fundamental surgical principle of immediate debridement of necrotic tissue and primary wound closure. Until recently, burns have always been the exception to this fundamental principle. With the ability of topical agents to control burn wound sepsis, topical therapy dominated burn treatment. Although the benefit to the patient by way of control of burn wound sepsis was enormous, it is well to recognize that this control was at the cost of slower spontaneous formation of burn eschar and, perhaps more importantly, an unstated philosophy implying that dead tissue produced by burning must be allowed to demarcate spontaneously before removal and that wound closure by skin graft must be carried out only after the development of a clean granulating recipient bed, thus resulting in a prolonged time between injury and wound closure. The past 10 years have seen the development of safe and effective blood replacement, improved monitoring equipment and, importantly, an understanding of the nutritional requirements of the thermally injured patient. The early excision and grafting of the burn wound have dramatically changed traditional burn care; however, this change has only been accepted slowly.

Early removal of large areas of full thickness burn to reduce the mortality and morbidity associated with thermal injuries has been attempted with varying degrees of success during the past 50 years. In 1929, following the successful application of excision in the management of gunshot wounds, Wells reported the use of primary excision in electrical burns, closures being primary or delayed.[1] In 1942, Young successfully excised a large area of full thickness burn of the back on the day of burning and immediately closed the wound with skin grafts.[2] The patient was discharged on the seventeenth hospital day. Cope in 1947 reported ten patients treated by surgical excision within three to five days following thermal injury. While the largest of these grafted areas was only 3% of the total body surface area (%TBSA), good graft take and effective closure of the burn wound was noted in 90% of the cases.[3] In 1953, McDowell emphasized the importance of early closure of excised wounds as a method of decreasing scar contractures which were frequently noted when granulating wounds were grafted.[4] In 1956, Meeker and Snyder reported their experience with dermatome debridement of burn wounds ranging from 15 to 65% TBSA in a group of 13 children.[5] Debridement of full thickness wounds with a dermatome resulted in earlier grafting, more rapid closure of the wound, and a reduction in the period of hospitalization, compared to a similar group of children treated by conventional therapy. MacMillan and Artz in 1957 reported their early experience in a prospective evaluation of early excision of 25% TBSA or more between the second and fifth days post-burn, and detailed the formidable nature of the procedures.[6]

Jackson in 1960, in a large controlled series of cases, found no conclusive evidence of a decrease in mortality rate or incidence of infection resulting from excisional procedures involving full thickness burns of 20 to 30% TBSA.[7] With the introduction of effective topical chemotherapeutic agents, Sulfamylon and silver nitrate, excision of the burn wound enjoyed little popularity. Moreover, Switzer in 1965 noted a high mortality rate in children treated by excision of areas of full thickness burn ranging from 20 to 50% TBSA.[8] In 1967, Bruce MacMillan at the Cincinnati Shriners Burns Institute, although a champion of primary excision and grafting for paediatric burns, reported no influence on mortality rate or incidence of septicaemia in wounds of 25% TBSA.[9] However, when excisional procedures were performed on areas of less than 15% of the body surface area, a significant improvement in post-operative morbidity was noted.

The development of the Tanner–Vanderput mesh dermatome facilitated skin grafting on excised beds because serum and blood could drain through the interstices of the meshed skin. In 1969, Haynes reported that with early excision and immediate or delayed grafting, the best results were obtained with excisional procedures of only 15% TBSA or less.[10] Zora Janzekovic, a Yugoslavian plastic surgeon, reported on the concept of tangential excision of deep dermal burn wounds.[11] Serial slices of burned tissue were excised until profuse bleeding was encountered; after haemostasis was obtained, split thickness autografts were applied. This was in contrast to the usual excisional procedures of excising down to deep fascia with a scalpel or a Bovie (diathermy), thus excising burned skin and subcutaneous tissue together. Between 1961 and 1974, Janzeko-vic treated 2615 burn patients with this form of tangential excision and sheet autografting.[12] Most of the burns were small, being less than 20%. However, dramatic decreases in hospital stay, pain, and number of reconstructive procedures were reported. Multiple authors, including Jackson and Stone in 1972,[13] Monafo in 1972,[14] Stone and Lawrence in 1973,[15] and Burke in 1974,[16] all reported decreased hospital stay and decrease in burn morbidity with the use of excisional therapy. Despite these impressive results, primary wound closure remained controversial even in the late 1970s.

In the early 1980s, more clinical and experimental data suggested better results and improved metabolic response following prompt wound closure. There was general agreement that small full thickness burns could be safely excised and grafted with good results and a shortened hospital stay, but the issue of deep dermal burns had not been resolved by a true prospective randomized trial. Heimbach at the University of Washington demonstrated that early excision and grafting of deep dermal burns of less than 20% TBSA resulted in decreased hospital stay, lower hospital costs, and less need for major reconstruction.[17] Furthermore, the excised group returned to work twice as fast as the non-operative group. Impressively, Heimbach demonstrated that after the adoption of early excision, the average stay was halved.

It is more difficult to prove that early excision improves survival with patients with extensive burns and in the elderly. These burns are fre-quently complicated by smoke inhalation, which adds a major variable in regard to survival. In addition, the elderly patient presents a unique problem in regard to survival. The atrophic skin of the elderly heals less successfully both in burn wounds and in donor sites. Moreover, they frequently present with co-morbid diseases such as cardiac pathology and diabetes.

With experience, early excision and grafting has become commonplace and is currently the treatment of choice for all deep dermal and full thickness burns. The procedure is still restricted by difficulty in diagnos-ing burn depth, by limited donor sites and technical skills to excise difficult areas such as the perineum and central portion of the face.

Selection of patients

The selection of patients for excisional therapy depends upon several factors including age, extent and depth of burn, interval between injury and initial examination, location of burn, presence of associated injury and illness, and, very importantly, adequate support facilities. Superficial burns that heal within two to three weeks will heal without hypertrophic scarring. These injuries result in no functional or cosmetic impairment after wound maturation. There may be an alteration in pigment from the surrounding skin and avoidance of direct exposure to the sun must be emphasized. Burns that benefit from early excision and grafting are the deep dermal burns and full thickness injury. Obvious full thickness injuries do not present a problem, in that they will all necessitate skin grafting if they are greater than 2.5 cm or they involve a critical area of the body. The sooner they can be grafted, the sooner wound coverage can be achieved. The deep dermal burns represent a more difficult problem, since depth of injury is difficult to determine. Despite multiple reports using various techniques, there is no consistently reliable device or laboratory test for measuring burn depth. Thus, the surgical diagnosis must be based upon surgical experience. The aetiology of the burn, inspection and palpation of the wound, and sensory functions are all useful in the diagnosis of depth of injury. Scald burns represent an even more difficult problem, in that they may be pink or bright red instead of white. These wounds, however, do not blanch with pressure and are generally not painful. Deep dermal burns heal with unstable epithelium, marked contracture formation and hypertrophic scarring.

If the injury is of indeterminate depth and is of small total body surface area, waiting as long as two weeks may be necessary to determine whether these wounds will heal. Frequently this can be accomplished on an outpatient basis, depending on the social status of the patient.

It is important to emphasize that of the major advances in burn management during the past 20 years, excision and grafting of deep dermal burns probably heads the list in regard to decreased hospital stay and rapid return to meaningful employment.

Pre-operative preparation

In major thermal injuries involving greater than 25% of the total body surface area, excisional therapy is usually delayed until after burn shock resuscitation is complete. This generally will require 48 hours. Herndon, at the Galveston Shriners Burns Institute, has reported remarkable results with massive excisions during the first 24 hours following extensive thermal injury.[18] In selection of the area, as a general rule, excision must be limited to 15 to 25% TBSA. If the surgical plan for a particular patient necessitates more than one procedure, critical areas must be grafted first to achieve optimum cosmetic and functional results. The order of preference for excisional procedures in extensive burns is the upper extremities, face, lower extremities, anterior trunk, and, finally, the back. Blood loss is a major consideration in excisional therapy, and in general approximately 200 ml per %TBSA burn excised and grafted will be required for excisional procedures.[19] In paediatric procedures, approximately 2% of the circulating blood volume per %TBSA burn excised and grafted will be needed. The optimum outcome from excisional and grafting procedures requires an experienced surgical and anaesthetic team. Excellent monitoring, nursing, physical and occupational therapy, nutritional support, and 24-hour experienced surgical and physician coverage are mandatory. Smaller burns in critical areas, such as the hands, face, feet and perineum, must be referred to a facility with experience in grafting such areas.

Surgical technique

Excision can be performed by fascial excision or layered excision. Fascial excision includes removing the burn and subcutaneous tissue to a level of the investing fascia. Fascial excision results in a viable graft bed, but frequently sacrifices viable fat and lymphatics, and results in an unacceptable cosmetic defect. The use of tourniquets may decrease blood loss. The use of a scalpel to remove the block of tissue is preferred, although electrocautery has been used successfully. Layered excision results in a significant blood loss, but leads to far superior results than fascial excision. The principle of layered excision is to shave very thin layers (0.002–0.003 inch) of burn eschar sequentially until viable tissue is reached. The procedure requires considerable experience and excellent operating room support. The technique can be accomplished with various instruments including the Padgett electric dermatome (Fig. 11.1), the Watson knife, or the Goulian knife (Fig. 11.2). If the bed does not bleed briskly, another slice at the same depth is taken until a viable bed of dermis or subcutaneous fat is reached. With experience, tourniquets may be utilized. When learning the technique, the tourniquet must be let down frequently to ensure an adequate graft bed. If there is a dull grey

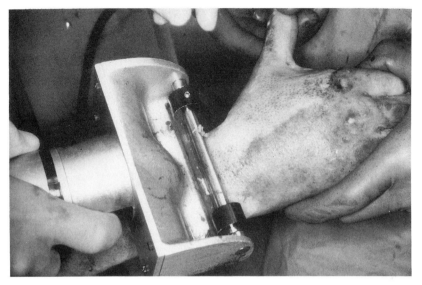

Fig. 11.1. Excision of dorsum of hand using Padgett dermatome.

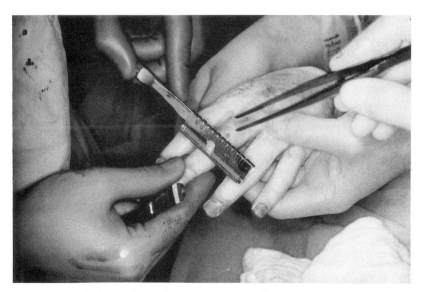

Fig. 11.2. Excision of fingers using Goulian knife.

appearance on the excised surface, or if there is evidence of clotted vessels, excision must be carried out more deeply. Facilitation of the excisional procedure can be accomplished by injecting saline solution with or without adrenaline (epinephrine) in a 1:50 000 solution. This technique results in decreased blood loss and creates a flat, firm surface facilitating excision of non-viable tissue. Bleeding is controlled with hot, adrenaline-soaked sponges and Bovie (diathermy) coagulation. The excised area can be wrapped for 10 to 15 minutes with Ace or crepe bandages to facilitate clotting.

In small burns, grafting may be accomplished on the same day as excision; however, the author's procedure is to use a two-stage method, with excision on one day, covering the excised wounds with a bulky gauze dressing soaked with an antibiotic/saline solution. If excision is accomplished without pneumatic tourniquets, bleeding is first controlled with hot compresses and adrenaline solution. If tourniquets were used, dressings are applied before tourniquet release. Dressings are held in place with gauze wraps and elastic bandages. The patient is then returned to the burn unit for recovery and wound care. Immediate attention is directed to restoration of normal body temperature, which can be achieved with radiant heat lamps, heat shields, thermal blankets, or warm water mattresses. Transfusions are given as necessary to maintain a haematocrit of 35% and normal blood volume. Excised wounds are kept moist by soaking dressings through irrigating catheters every four hours. On the following day, the patient is returned to the operating room for skin graft coverage of the excised burns. Split thickness autografts are taken with a Padgett electric dermatome at a thickness of 0.008 to 0.016 inch. To facilitate harvesting of autograft, subcutaneous tissue is distended with an infusion of Ringer's lactate using a roller pump apparatus (Fig. 11.3). Adrenaline may be added to the Ringer's solution (1:10 000) to help control bleeding. While skin for grafting is excised, dressings are removed from the excised wounds and bleeding is controlled with hot adrenaline-soaked sponges and Bovie electrocautery coagulation. Major bleeding sites are ligated.

Meshed skin grafts have been extensively utilized with early excision and grafting techniques. In extensive burns greater than 60% total body surface area, frequently 1:4 meshed skin is utilized. Previously, almost all small burns were grafted with meshed skin expanded to a ration of 1:1.5 or 1:3. Although this technique yields acceptable cosmetic results compared to older skin graft techniques, the meshed pattern still is cosmetically unacceptable. Sheet grafts must be utilized in burns of less than 40%

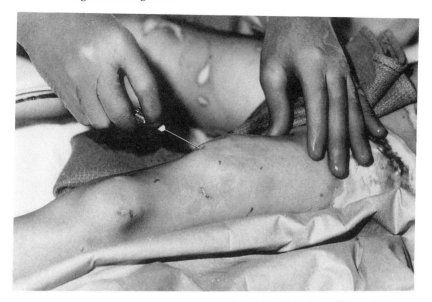

Fig. 11.3. Distention of skin of thigh with an infusion of Ringer's lactate using a roller pump apparatus to facilitate harvesting of autograft.

total body surface area. In burns of 40 to 60%, sheet autograft is utilized on the hands and face, with expanded grafts on the other areas. This has given a more acceptable cosmetic result and a marked decrease in wound maturation time. The length of time of wearing pressure dressings is decreased 50% with the use of sheet grafts.

Freshly applied autografts are dressed with fine mesh gauze, and covered with bulky dressings and irrigating catheters. Extremities are splinted with Hexolite splints and elastic bandages. Patients are returned to the burn unit, where attention is given to temperature control, blood volume replacement and analgesia. The skin grafts are soaked through irrigating catheters every 4 hours with an antibiotic solution, either DAB solution (neomycin sulphate 40mg/l, polymyxin B 200 μg/l), or a 2.5% solution of Sulfamylon, depending upon the flora of the burn wound (Fig. 11.4).[19] After 48 hours the dressings are removed and the wounds are examined. Skin grafts are then redressed with bulky dressings for an additional three days. On the fifth post-grafting day, the staples are removed and the grafts are covered with a light layer of bacitracin ointment, covered with a layer of non-adherent gauze, and wrapped with gauze rolls. Active range of motion exercise of the grafted areas is begun on the fifth day post-grafting. If sheet autograft is utilized, the wounds can

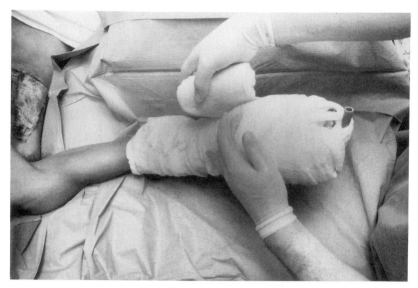

Fig. 11.4. Post skin grafting dressing consisting of fine mesh gauze, bulky burn dressings, Kerlix and Ace bandages. Irrigating catheters are utilized to keep wounds moist.

generally be placed in a moisturizing cream on the seventh post-grafting day. If meshed graft is utilized, the wounds are kept in bacitracin ointment until the epithelium migrates across the interstices of the mesh graft.

Specialized areas

Face

Restoration of the burned face remains one of the greatest challenges in the management of burn patients. Burns of the head and neck region occur in over 50% of patients admitted with thermal injury and frequently result in devastating alterations in cosmetic appearance. Although surgical management of burn wounds, with aggressive early excision and immediate skin graft coverage, has become increasingly widespread in burn centres, management of the face burn has remained conservative, allowing deep dermal wounds to heal and full-thickness burns to form granulation tissue before skin grafting.

Indications for excisional therapy of burns of the face and neck include:

1. obvious full-thickness injury,
2. burn wounds not healed by 14 days post-injury or
3. absence of 'epithelial buds' in the wound at 14 days post-burn.[20]

Excision and grafting of facial burns is performed in a two-day procedure. General anaesthesia is induced with an oral or nasotracheal tube secured either by suturing to the teeth or by packing the mouth tightly with gauze sponges. The subcutaneous tissue beneath the burn is infiltrated with Ringer's lactate solution containing adrenaline (1:50 000). Volumes ranging from a few millilitres to 500–600 ml of solution are used, depending on the extent of injury and facial area involved. Distention of subcutaneous tissue greatly decreases bleeding and facilitates excision of the burn wound by flattening convex and contoured areas of the face. Wounds are excised using either a small hand (Goulian) or electric dermatome set to remove layers of eschar at a thickness of 0.014 inch or until a viable layer is reached. Excised wounds are covered with bulky gauze dressings soaked with saline. On the day following excision, patients are returned to the operating room for autograft coverage of the excised wounds. Donor sites are selected for best colour match, and moderately thick split-thickness autografts are harvested with the electric dermatome at a thickness of 0.018 to 0.024 inch. The scalp has become the primary donor site for initial coverage of large excised wounds of the face and neck. The use of subcutaneous infiltration of Ringer's lactate greatly facilitates harvesting skin from the scalp. The neck or infraclavicular donor site regions are usually preserved for late reconstructive procedures. The skin grafts are held in position with staples, covered with a light layer of bacitracin ointment and left open. Postoperatively, the grafts are rolled hourly to remove serum collection.

Technically, excisional procedures of the face are extremely difficult, with massive blood loss and difficulty in removing non-viable tissue in the contoured areas of the central face. Blood loss for excision and grafting procedures of the face and neck averages 500 ml per %TBSA.[20] Post-operative application of pressure devices is imperative. A duplicate model of the face is made 7 to 10 days postoperatively, and a clear plastic face mask is made from the mould.

Hands and upper extremities

The same philosophy of excisional therapy pertains to hand burns as to other areas of the body.[21] Unless the hands are charred, excision is always

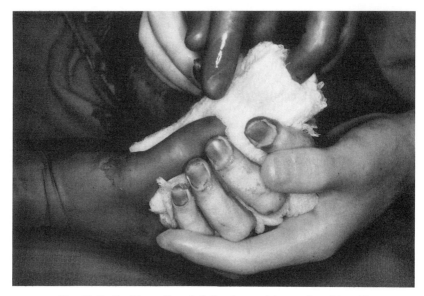

Fig. 11.5. Position of hands following excision and grafting. Fingers are wrapped around a Kerlix roll and wrapped in bulky wet dressings.

performed using the layered or sequential technique. A tourniquet is utilized; however, the tourniquet may be let down if depth of excision is questionable. The oedema of burn shock will facilitate excision. The Padgett electric dermatome is used for the dorsum of the hand and a Goulian knife for the fingers. The dorsum of the hand is excised first followed by the fingers and thumb. Towel clips are utilized to stabilize the finger during the excisional procedure. The two-stage technique is utilized in all but the very small burns. Towel clips placed through the fingertips and hung on a holder facilitate graft placement. The grafts are held in position with the use of staples. During the excisional procedure, the dorsal hood of the proximal interphalangeal joint (PIP) must be examined carefully. Postoperatively, the hand is placed in position of function with a Kerlix roll placed in the palm and wet dressings applied as above. There is no need to place the PIP joint in extension if the dorsal hood is not damaged. Placing the fingers in a curved position facilitates the rehabilitative process (Fig. 11.5).[22] The wounds are cared for as described above, with early range of motion exercises on the fifth postoperative day. If the dorsal hood of the PIP is destroyed, K-wire pins are utilized to maintain position of function of the joint and prevent Boutonnière deformity.

Trunk and perineum

The perineum and trunk are difficult areas to which to apply a dressing. The use of back donor sites frequently necessitates wrapping these areas. Spandex material stapled over bulky dressings, incorporating the irrigating catheters, facilitates grafting these areas. The patient can be rolled and donor sites can be cared for properly.

Donor sites

In the past, donor sites were covered with either dry fine-mesh gauze, or gauze impregnated with a dye or other antimicrobial agent. They were left to desiccate and the gauze generally separated from the wound in 2 to 3 weeks, frequently removing new epithelium with it. Major thermal burns which have donor sites adjacent to unexcised burns or grafted areas are treated as second degree burns utilizing bacitracin (Adaptic) with twice-daily dressing changes. Although still necessitating twice-a-day washing, this method has resulted in no infections nor conversion to full thickness donor site wounds. In smaller burns, Biobrane may be utilized. This has the advantages of no dressing changes and decreased pain, but it must be stapled into position.[23] Other techniques include adhesive polyurethane sheets;[24] however, there must be a margin of 3 to 4 cm of normal skin to allow the margins of the material to adhere. Donor sites are not free of complications. In addition to hypertrophic scarring and pigmentation, patients may experience blistering for several weeks. The blisters are generally self-limited and are treated with bandages or ointment until they re-epithelialize. Infections occur infrequently, and may be treated with systemic antibiotics or silver sulphadiazine.

Critical burns

Although excisional therapy is well accepted and has given excellent results in small to moderate burns, in the extensively burned patient in which donor sites are limited and in which wound closure cannot be accomplished early in the burn treatment period, several techniques are available. Most burn surgeons still feel that early removal of the non-viable eschar is essential and coverage may be accomplished by several methods. If a homograft skin bank is available, then fresh homograft applied to the excised wound will buy valuable time. In addition, Biobrane has been demonstrated to be as useful as frozen homograft in maintaining a temporary coverage.[25] The early work using the artificial dermis developed by Burke in Boston shows promise but is still in the developmental stage.[26,27] The use of cultured epidermal cells, although enjoying popularity, results in hypertrophic scarring and extremely unstable epithelium. Although the use of cultured epidermal cells may be useful in massively burned patients with burns of greater than 85 to 90% of the total body surface area, this technique for wound coverage necessitates further experimental work to develop a true coverage for these massively burned patients.[28]

Rehabilitation

Although excisional procedures have dramatically decreased the hospital stay and have improved the cosmetic results in thermally injured patients, the use of pressure dressings and active range of motion exercises, proper use of splinting techniques and clear pressure face masks are of utmost importance to achieve the final result. Incorporation of the rehabilitation team into the total care of the burn patient is mandatory. The technique of excisional therapy is only one aspect of the surgical management of the burn patient. Experienced support members of the burn team, including nursing staff, rehabilitation, social work, and nutrition, as well as the family members, are the key to successful surgical management of the burn patient.

References

1 Wells DB. The treatment of electric burns by immediate resection and skin graft. *Ann Surg* 1928; **90**:1069–78.
2 Young F. Immediate skin grafting in the treatment of burns. *Ann Surg* 1942; **116**:445–51.
3 Cope O, Laughohr J, Moore ED *et al.* Expeditious care of full thickness burn wounds by surgical excision and grafting. *Ann Surg* 1947; **125**:1–22.
4 Mcdowell F. Accelerated excision and grafting of small deep burns. *Am J Surg* 1953; **85**:407–10.
5 Meeker IA, Snyder WH. Dermatome debridement and early grafting of extensive third degree burns in children. *Surg Gyn Obst* 1956; **103**:527–34.
6 MacMillan BG, Artz CP. A planned evaluation of early excision of more than twenty-five percent of the body surface in burns. *Surg Forum* 1957; **7**:88–93.
7 Jackson D, Topley E, Cason JS *et al.* primary excision and grafting of large burns. *Ann Surg* 1960; **152**:167–89.
8 Switzer WE, Jones JW, Moncrief JA. Evaluation of early excision of burns in children. *J Trauma* 1965; **5**:540–6.
9 MacMillan BG. Wound management. Early excision. *J Trauma* 1967; **7**:75–9.
10 Haynes BW. Early excision and grafting in third degree burns. *Ann Surg* 1969; **169**:736–47.

11 Janzekovic Z. A new concept in the early excision and immediate grafting of burns. *J Trauma* 1970; **10**:1103–8.

12 Janzekovic Z. The burn wound from the surgical point of view. *J Trauma* 1975; **15**:42–62.

13 Jackson DM, Stone PA. Tangential excision and grafting of burns: the method and a report of 50 consecutive cases. *Br J Plast Surg* 1972; **25**:416–26.

14 Monafo WW, Aulenbacher CE, Pappalarado C. Early tangential excision of the eschars of major burns. *Arch Surg* 1972; **104**:503–8.

15 Stone PA, Lawrence JC. Healing of tengentially excised and grafted burns in man. *Br J Plast Surg* 1973; **26**:20–31.

16 Burke JF, Bondoc CC, Quinby WC. Primary burn excision and immediate grafting: a method shortening illness. *J Trauma* 1974; **144**:389–95.

17 Engrav LH, Heimbach DM, Reus JL, *et al.* Early excision and grafting vs. nonoperative treatment of burns of indeterminate depth: a randomized prospective study. *J Trauma* 1983; **23**:101–4.

18 Herndon DN, Barron RE, Rutan RL, Rutan TC, Desai MH, Abston S. A comparison of conservative versus early excision. *Ann Surg* 1989; **209**:547–52.

19 Warden GD, Saffle JR, Kravitz M: A two stage technique for excision and grafting of burn wounds. *J Trauma* 1982; **22**:98–102.

20 Warden GD, Saffle JR, Schnebly A, Kravitz M. Excisional therapy of facial burns. *J Burn Care & Rehabil* 1986; **7**:24–8.

21 Hunt JL, Sato R, Baxter CR. Early tangential excision and immediate mesh autografting of deep dermal hand burns. *Ann Surg* 1979; **189**:147–51.

22 Schnebly A, Kravitz M, Warden GD. Hand splinting in the 'natural' position of function: the method of choice following excision and grafting of thermally injured hands. *Proceedings Twelfth Annual Meeting American Burn Association*, San Antonio, Texas, 1980.

23 Zapata-Sirvent R, Hansbrough JF, Carroll W *et al.* Comparison of Biobrane and scarlet red dressings for treatment of donor site wounds. *Arch Surg* 1985; **120**:743–5.

24 James JH, Watson ACH. The use of Op-Site, a vapour permeable dressing, on skin graft donor sites. *Br J Plast Surg* 1975; **28**:107–10.

25 Purdue GF, Hunt JL, Gillespie RW *et al.* Biosynthetic skin substitute versus frozen cadaver allograft for temporary coverage of excised burn wounds. *J Trauma* 1987; **27**:155–7.

26 Burke JF, Yannas IV, Quinby WC *et al.* Successful use of a physiologically acceptable artificial skin in the treatment of extensive burn injury. *Ann Surg* 1981; **194**:413–28.

27 Heimbach D, Luterman A, Burke J *et al.* Artificial dermis for major burns: a multicenter randomized clinical trial. *Ann Surg* 1988; **208**:313–20.

28 Gallico GG, O'Connor NE, Compton CC *et al.* Permanent coverage of large burn wounds with autologous cultured human epithelium. *N Eng J Med* 1984; **311**:448–51.

12

Postoperative care of the burned patient

R. BUNSELL

Introduction

Postoperative care of the burned patient must fall to a team of health care workers who have been trained and are experienced in the management of this challenging clinical problem. Care is most appropriately given by a committed team which includes, amongst others, surgeons, anaesthetists, physicians, psychiatrists, pathology services, nurses, physiotherapists, occupational therapists, dieticians, medical social workers and chaplains. Wherever possible, the patients family must be involved in the care and rehabilitation.

The care must be afforded in a purpose-built unit in which temperature and humidity can be controlled, and where patients can be easily isolated if necessary. The unit must have the facility to receive patients and nurse them in a range of areas from one prepared for the whole spectrum of critical care to low dependency nursing areas.[1]

Post-operative management begins in the pre-operative period. If it is at all possible to communicate with the patient, they must be informed prior to going to the operating theatre of what will be done (informed consent) and what to expect regarding dressings and discomfort. Without being untruthful, this must be done with tact and in a reassuring manner. If it is planned to move the patient to another ward area in the post-operative period the patient and any family must be informed. Pre-operative visiting by the anaesthetist and by the recovery room staff must be mandatory.

Postanaesthetic recovery (PAR)

Admitting the patient to the PAR and later discharging the patient to the ward is the responsibility of the anaesthetist. Burn surgery is frequently

164

shocking, with major blood loss and body cooling. The patient will also have been given significant doses of opiate analgesics. Accordingly, the anaesthetist must be quite certain that the patient is close to normovolaemia, is breathing adequately, and has adequate analgesia before leaving the operating room.

Monitoring

The patient must be handed over to a trained recovery nurse, and accompanied to the PAR area. Oxygen must be administered in transfer and be continued in PAR.[2,3] Good nursing technique will ensure on arrival in PAR that the patient remains in an acceptable clinical state in recovery, with monitoring commencing quickly, and all vascular lines checked for security and function.

Monitoring in recovery must include a non invasive blood pressure (NIBP) machine, ECG and pulse oximetry. Monitors may also be used from theatre such as invasive pressure transducers, central venous manometry and urine output measurement.[4,5] Access to the patient is often limited due to dressings and splints and conventional monitoring may be very difficult. NIBP may well work through dressings; though the numbers generated may not be accurate they will still provide a trend which will be useful. Electrocardiography (ECG), if electrodes can be placed on the patient, will give rate, rhythm and wave form. (ECG is not a first line monitor since it will give little evidence of perfusion or oxygenation until the patient collapses.) Pulse oximetry is an excellent monitor giving rate, an indication of rhythm and perfusion as well as oxygen saturation. The numeric value of oxygen saturation may be erroneously high if the patient has been poisoned by carbon monoxide.[6] Ideally, where carbon monoxide inhalation has been suspected, the carboxyhaemoglobin level must be measured, but the adverse effect on oxygen saturation will be relevant only if the patient is taken to theatre in the first 36 hours, after which carbon monoxide will have been mostly eliminated if oxygen therapy has been used.

Invasive monitoring lines are not used for trivial reasons as they will increase the number of portals of entry for sepsis. However, if indicated, these lines (arterial and/or central venous cannulation with or without a flotation catheter) may be used. Such lines may be placed electively if massive transfusion is anticipated or if the anaesthetist 'loses his way' in managing the fluids using only non-invasive monitoring techniques. Introduction of lines with an aseptic technique in sites of election is a counsel of excellence which in practice may not be possible. Lines placed urgently in sub-optimal conditions must be replaced electively within 24 hours.

Measurement of haematological values in PAR and later in post-operative management must be used with great caution. Clotting studies in the presence of continued blood loss are useful and permit the rational use of blood component therapy guided by a haematologist. In the acute setting values of haemoglobin and haematocrit can be associated with an unacceptable error leading to overload or under transfusion.[7] There remains a place for clinical skills to estimate optimal fluid replacement.

Urine output must be maintained at 0.5ml/kg/h. Oliguria at this time is almost invariably due to hypovolaemia. Hypovolaemia must be treated with fluid replacement, preferably with a blood product or other colloid. Rapid bolus administration is the most satisfactory method of rendering the patient volume replete. Modest increases in a fluid infusion is usually a slow and inadequate method of correcting hypovolaemia. Syringing fluid into the patient through a dry infusion warming device is rapid and effective but must only be done by a member of the medical staff. The use of diuretics such as Frusemide must be avoided. (Their use must only be sanctioned by the senior anaesthetist when indicated.)

Analgesia

The value of adequate analgesia from the PAR continuing onto the ward cannot be overstated. Leaving a patient in agony is an anaesthetic failure which can adversely affect the outcome of the operation. A distressed agitated patient can easily detach the recently applied split skin grafts even under substantial dressings.[8] It is acknowledged that paediatric patients are usually under treated with analgesic drugs.[9] Analgesia will have been addressed intra-operatively and its efficacy must be assessed by the anaesthetist in PAR. Short acting synthetic opioids such as fentanyl or alfentanil are most elegantly used by infusion, in which case the infusion may be continued in the postoperative period.[10] Longer acting opiates such as the alkaloid papaveretum may be chosen as the intra-operative and postoperative analgesic. In recovery, if the patient is distressed the anaesthetist must titrate an intravenous dose of opiate to render the patient comfortable. Intramuscular doses must not be used as adminis-tration may be technically very difficult in the heavily bandaged patient, and absorption from the injection site cannot be predicted. These reasons also mitigate against intramuscular analgesics in many patients later in their management on the ward. Opiate analgesic infusions therefore offer high-quality analgesia in many burned patients. Patient-controlled analgesia (PCA)[11] offers an excellent infusion technique provided the patient has been instructed in the use of the device pre-operatively, is co-operative enough, and has one hand capable of operating the sensor hand piece. PCA does not require a 'background infusion' rate since this does not help the quality of analgesia, but only increases morbidity.[12] Frequently, however, one or more of the criteria is not met in which case a continuous infusion from a syringe driver will have to be used.[13] Opiate infusions of this type may be fraught with problems of safety.[14] They may only be used in areas where there are adequate numbers of trained nurses experienced in their use. All staff must be aware of the risk of somnolence, and respiratory depression. Considerable co-operation between the anaesthetist and the nurse is imperative. A protocol of use must be established so that the dose given is monitored as well as its effect: an explicitly written dose regime with a range of rates such that the bedside nurse can, with experience, safely alter the rate to suit the needs of the patient. At the first suspicion of respiratory depression, the infusion must be stopped, and an appropriate member of the medical team called. Naloxone must always be available. If, for logistic reasons, there is an inadequate number of trained and experienced staff to supervise an opiate infusion then it must not be used. In this situation intermittent intra-muscular doses of opiate will have to be used. Intra-muscular dosing may be made more tolerable, especially in the child, if at the time of operation a fine bore inert plastic intravenous cannula is placed and secured in the deltoid muscle (Wallace Y-can 23G). This will permit less painful intra-muscular drug administration. If control of analgesia is lost in the PAR the inhalation of Entonox will give respite until the anaesthetist can attend and give intravenous analgesia.

Nutrition

Nutritional support must be established as soon as is practical. If nothing else in patients with burns in excess of 15% TBSA a small bore soft nasogastric feeding tube (clinifeed tube) must be placed. If not already in place this is most kindly done at the time of the first operation. Checking placement of the tube by means of a radiograph may be requested in PAR. If a feeding enterostomy has been inserted, its security and patency must be checked.

Only when the anaesthetist is satisfied that the patient is breathing well, oxygenated, comfortable and adequately resuscitated from operative losses can the patient be allowed to return to the burns ward.

Ward care

Analgesia

In the ward area, the postoperative patient will require analgesic management as outlined in the PAR section for some two days until the donor sites and other painful areas are less sore. Surgeons must be encouraged at the time of operation to use contemporary dressings such as Kaltostat (TM), Biobrane (TM) or a polyurethane cover which will reduce the pain from donor sites. Dressing changes and other manoeuvres can be agonizing, and anticipation of further painful events can have a profoundly depressing effect on the patient. The service of a trained and experienced anaesthetist to render the patient 'analgesic' during painful dressing changes is invaluable. As nutrition is vital to the healing (and survival of the patient)[15] no technique must be used which leaves the patient unable to eat or absorb food for long periods of time. Opiates and Ketamine have been used, but the judicious use of Propofol offers the patient insensibility and very rapid recovery and remains the best available management of the patient's pain during dressings. Results of this technique require a skilled anaesthetist able to manage any possible complications. Many burns units will not have an anaesthetist available for dressings, and analgesia will then fall to self administered Entonox (TM) or volatile agent inhalers (enflurane or isoflurane). This requires commitment from the nursing staff to whom special training must be given.

Nutrition

Virtually no patient with a serious burn will be able to eat and drink a sufficient diet to heal. Malnourishment is associated with an increased risk of morbidity and mortality from sepsis as the patients immune system is very sensitive to poor nutrition. Nutritional support may be enteral (much the preferred technique) or parenteral.[16-20]

Enteral feeding may be oral, nasogastric or by feeding enterostomy. The latter permits feeding even in the presence of gastric stasis.

Parenteral feeding may be peripheral or central. Peripheral feeding is limited by the amount of calories and nitrogen which can be given, and also peripheral veins are at a premium in the burned patient. Central feeding by means of a dedicated feeding line which has been tunnelled permits more calories and nitrogen to be given. Surgeons at the time of surgery must always be encouraged to excise and graft any burns which

involve sites of election (e.g. infraclavicular areas) for central cannulation in the event that line insertion is required later for feeding or
monitoring. A calorie to nitrogen ratio of 150:1 must be used and the
feeds modified to the patients actual needs. Nitrogen losses should be
calculated.(See Chapter on Nutrition)

Monitoring effectiveness of therapy will rely mainly on serum albumin
measurements with assays of trace elements. Parameters such as body
weight and skin fold thickness may not be possible in many patients.

Physical therapy

The essence of treatment of all patients involves the return of function
and rehabilitation. Physiotherapy and occupational therapy are therefore
an integral part of management. Chest physiotherapy will be therapeutic
in the management of some patients with respiratory problems and may
prevent or reduce complications such as secretion retention and infection. To this end, minitracheostomy may be used.[21,22] When wound
healing permits, active and passive movement of joints assumes a high
priority. Occupational therapists skilled in the management of the burn
injured hand are important team members. Early application of sophisticated splints may improve hand function on healing. It is worth emphasis-
ing a principle of trauma management, that when dealing with life-
threatening injury, meticulous attention to small details will permit the
patient a better quality of survival. Areas of attention, sadly often
neglected, are the hands, feet and eyes.[23]

Psychological aspects

Up to 50% of adult burned patients have psychiatric disorders ranging
from tobacco smoking to major psychoses, including the dementias and
drug and alcohol abuse.[24] The assistance of a psychiatrist can only serve
to improve their management whilst an inpatient. An affective disorder
related to the injury and its consequences is not pathological and must be
dealt with by all the staff involved showing compassionate realism. Here,
the role of the psychiatrist can be used in the 'grand round' and take the
form of educating the conventional burns staff, and the value of the
medical social worker (MSW) can also be shown. They may be able to
bring insight into cultural or social problems associated with the injury.
The significance of non-accidental injury in children must not be

overstated, but staff will be expected to have a high level of suspicion and training by the MSW will be helpful.

It is common, and perhaps invariable, for the families of burned adults and especially burned children to suffer guilt.[25] This guilt can be incapacitating, inducing illness in some family members. This is particularly true if the patient dies. Accordingly, every unit must have a form of counselling service for families which can include any of the team, though here again a psychiatrist and MSW have an obvious role, as does the chaplaincy service. In making provision for management of stress, the need for support of staff members must not be forgotten.[26] Important features of those involved in counselling are as follows.

1. Compassionate honesty
2. Experience based on counselling training
3. Efficiency in following up groups at risk
4. Willingness to include other agencies and family practitioners.

Complications

Complications of burn care are legion. The following are dealt with in separate chapters and are mentioned here only briefly.

1. Fluid management.
2. Renal failure may be precipitated by hypovolaemia, sepsis, other injuries and severe electrical burns (due to release of myoglobin[27]). Renal failure may be managed by spontaneous or machine driven haemofiltration. If the patient is very catabolic, however, dialysis may be required. There is no place for peritoneal dialysis. Wherever possible renal failure must be attended to in an area where the primary injury will not be neglected.
3. Anaemia.
4. Sepsis; systemic antibiotics must always be guided by microbiologists, requiring frequent culture swabs and blood cultures when indicated. There is a place for topical antibiotics, e.g. silver sulphadiazine.[28] The value of selective digestive tract decontamination may prove promising.[29]
5. Respiratory failure may be due to a primary insult from inhaled toxic smoke or from systemic sepsis. These patients will require ventilation. Patients may also require more than one flexible fibre-optic bronchoscopy and indeed fibre-optic laryngoscopy

may be in skilled hands, the safest way to intubate the burned patient who has upper airway swelling.

6. Pruritus in the healing phase can be very distressing. The itching has features similar to the pruritus due to neuraxial opiates. Naloxone, nalbuphine and buprenorphine has been used empirically with good effect.[30]

References

1 Anonymous. Facilities for burns treatment in the UK. *Burns* 1978; **4**:297.
2 Demling RH, Lalonde C. Oxygen consumption is increased in the post-anaesthetic period after burn excision. *J Burn Care & Rehabil* 1989; **10(5)**:381.
3 Jones JG, Sapsford DJ, Wheatley RG. Post operative hypoxaemia. *Br J Anaesth* 1990; **45**:566.
4 Sykes MK. Essential monitoring. *Br J Anaesth* 1987; **59**:901.
5 Eichorn JH, Cooper D, Cullen DJ *et al*. Standards for patient monitoring during anaesthesia at Harvard Medical School. *J Am Med Assn* 1986; **256**:1017.
6 Petty TL. *Clinical Pulse Oximetry*. Webb-Waring Lung Institute, Denver, Colorado, 1986.
7 Shoemaker WC, Kram HB. Crystalloid and colloid therapy in resuscitation and subsequent I.C.U. management. *Clin Anaesthesiol* 1988; **2(3)**:509.
8 Wall PD. The prevention of postoperative pain. *Pain* 1988; **33**:289–90.
9 Lloyd Thomas AR. Pain management in paediatric patients. *Br J Anaesth* 1990; **64**:85–104.
10 Mitchell RW, Smith G. The control of acute postoperative pain. *Br J Anaesth* 1989; **63**:147.
11 Rosen M. P.C.A. in practice. *Seminars in Anaesthesia* 1986; **5**:108.
12 Notcutt. Developing the use of P.C.A. in a District General Hospital. In: *The Edinburgh Symposium on Pain Control and Medical Education*. RSM Internat Congress & Symposium Series. 1989.
13 Bollish SJ, Collins CL, Kirking DM. Efficacy of P.C.A. versus conventional analgesia for post-op pain. *Clin Pharm* 1985; **4**:48–52.
14 White PF. Mishaps with P.C.A. *Anaesthesiology* 1987; **66**:81–3.
15 Henley M. Feed that burn. *Burns* 1989; **15(6)**:351–61.
16 King N, Goodwin Jr CW. Use of vitamin supplements for burned patients. *J Am Diet Assn* 1984; **8**:923–5.
17 Bell SW, Wyatt J. Nutritional guidelines for burned patients. *J Am Diet Assn* 1986; **5**:648–53.
18 Pasulka PS, Watchel TL. Nutritional considerations for the burned patient. *Surg Clin N Am* 1987; **67(1)**:109–31.
19 Herndon DN, *et al*. Increase mortality with I.V. supplemental feeding in severely burned patients. *J Burn Care & Rehabil* 1989; **10(4)**:309.
20 Klasen HJ, ten Duis HJ. Early oral feeding of patients with extensive burns. *Burns* 1987; **13(1)**:49–52.
21 Mathews HR, Hopkinson RB. Treatment of sputum retention by mini tracheostomy. *Br J Surg* 1984; **71**:147–50.

22 Randel T, Kalli I, Lindgren L. Mini tracheostomy; complications and follow up with tracheoscopy. *Anaesthesia* 1990; **45**:875.
23 London PS. Personal communication. Senior Surgeon Birmingham Accident Hospital. 1991.
24 Roberts AHN. Personal communication. Director Burns Unit, Stoke Mandeville Hospital. 1991.
25 Scrubby LS, Sloan JA. Bereavement, counselling, family, home care. *Can J Pub Health* 1989; **80(6)**:394–8.
26 Cathcart F. Dealing with stress. *Nursing Times* 1989; **85(43)**:33–5.
27 Luce EA, Gottlieb SE. True high tension electrical injuries. *Inn Plast Surg* 1984; **12**:321–6.
28 Livingstone DH, Cryer HG, Miller FB, *et al.* Topical antimicrobial agents on skin grafts after thermal injury. *Plast & Reconstr Surg* 1990; **86(6)**:1059–64.
29 Ledingham I McA, Alcock SR, Eastaway AT *et al.* Selective digestive tract decontamination. *Lancet* 1988; **i**:785.
30 Rylah LTA. Personal communication. Director of Critical Care, Billericay Burns Unit. 1991.

13

Prognosis of the burn injury

A.D. WILMSHURST

Introduction

Survival or death following a burn is highly dependent on the age of the victim and the extent of the injury. Other factors play lesser though important roles, and ultimate survival depends on successful management of the patient both initially and through the course of a number of potential complications. As a measure of success, the mortality rate is the most important, the most easily quantified and the only unequivocal outcome parameter. Crude mortality figures, however, are of little value. They must be related to the factors that are known to influence prognosis. It is an examination of these severity factors and the weight which various authorities have assigned to them that occupies this chapter. Simple techniques and systems which enable one to estimate prognosis in the individual case or to compare performance within or between burn units will also be discussed.

Historical aspect

From the early years of the twentieth century it has been recognized that survival of a burn is related to the proportion of body surface burned and the age of the patient. However, a numerical definition of this relationship was not proposed until 1949 when Bull and Squire[1] presented an approximate mortality probability grid, derived by probit analysis based on their experience of 794 burn patients. Bull revised this work in 1954,[2] and again in 1971,[3] including further experience and figures reflecting generally improved survival. Since Bull's first publication a number of workers have identified additional characteristics of burned patients which have significant bearing upon their survival. Increasingly sophisticated statistical techniques have been applied to expanding series of patients. Some of the most valuable contributions have come from groups pooling data from a number of burn centres; the well documented work from the National Burn Information Exchange (NBIE) in North America is a prime example.[4-8] Provided a valid statistical analysis can be made on a sufficient number of patients on survival in the presence of documented risk factors, predictions may then follow on the probability that a given patient will, or will not, survive the injury.

Following a period of apparent near stagnation in burn management and survival rates during the middle decades of this century, the past 25 years have seen major advances in burn care with a concurrent improvement in survival.[9-12] The specific reasons for the rise in survival rates may be more subtle than some writers suggest. Although it is universally agreed that age and per cent total body surface area (%TBSA) burned are two of the most important, there is a variety of severity factors involved in the burned patient which may affect the final prognosis.

Factors present before the injury

Age

Bull and Squire[1] in their pioneering paper in 1949, were able to state that 'age . . . .as is well known, has a very marked effect on the outcome of a burn'. Since that time, every severity index or model proposed has included the age of the patient as a fundamental element. It is now well established that, for a given size of burn the prognosis worsens with advancing years after early adult life. There is some controversy over survival rates in early life. Bull's studies, which were notable for very large numbers in the age group 0 to 5 years, produced mortality curves showing little change up to the age of 30. Several other large series [13-16] have clearly demonstrated a worse prognosis in very young children. This is attributed generally to the immaturity of the immune system and repair mechanisms at this age.

Survival falls markedly after the age of 50: a typical report in 1980 gives figures for the LA50 (lethal area of burn for 50% of the burn population) as 71.2% in the 5–34 year age group reducing to 19.6% in those over 75 years.

Sex

Most studies that have included an analysis of the influence of sex on mortality have reported a positive correlation, mortality being higher in females.[4,15-17] The relationship is never particularly strong, and it must be noted that two other reports, both from large series in individual burn centres[14,18] failed to show an association. A possible explanation of the positive correlation is that mortality is inversely related to the proportion of lean body mass. In support of this, Barrow and Herndon[19] have demonstrated that overweight boys are more likely to get burned, and that these boys have a significantly raised mortality rate.

Race

Sufficiently large series of patients with a racial mix to allow satisfactory comparison of survival data are few, and the results are conflicting. Where survival is reduced in a Negro population, it is more plausible that the difference is due to socioeconomic status rather than any genetic predisposition.[14]

Medical history

As in other forms of major trauma, the pre-existing health of the individual has a crucial bearing on the outcome of the burn injury. Severity and type of past medical history are clearly difficult to quantify when predicting its effect on prognosis. However, if the healthy elderly are considered as a distinct group from their counterparts with one or more recognized diseases, survival curves diverge significantly.[2] In the very large NBIE series, the authors were able to show that each past medical problem existing in a burn patient was equivalent to the effect of a burn injury of 11% TBSA.[12] Cardiorespiratory and circulatory conditions are particularly important. Baux[20] found that respiratory disease, peripheral and central vascular disease and severe hypertension were associated with a much higher mortality in an elderly group of patients.

Factors present as components of the injury

Area

The percentage of total body surface area burned remains as one of the factors most closely associated with mortality, even after extensive investigation into other severity factors by many authorities. The importance of area of burn was documented in the mid-1940s and Bull in 1949 subjected it to probit analysis to produce a linear relationship with mortality.

Area of full thickness burn

Due to the increased risk of sepsis and the demands placed upon the patient by surgery for wound closure, greater nutritional needs, and higher blood loss, a deep burn represents a considerably more severe injury in terms of prognosis than a partial thickness burn of the same area. Most burns of any extent are of mixed thickness, and there may be considerable difficulty in defining the full thickness areas on admission. For this reason, many published analyses have disregarded the area of full thickness burn. Where it has been included in statistical analysis, the effect of full thickness burn is generally found to be greater than that of partial thickness injury. A relative predictive value is sometimes assigned, giving deep burns between two and four times the value of the equivalent partial thickness burn.[1,20]

Site

The part of the body burned may have some bearing on prognosis if, for instance, it is associated with a higher risk of infection, or on the other hand reflects the external injury related to a respiratory burn. Thus Moores, reviewing the experience of the Yorkshire Regional Unit,[17] found that burns of the bathing trunk area ('pyo-prone' patients) had a significantly increased mortality. This has been confirmed by the NBIE surveys.[16] Burns to the face may also be associated with a poorer prognosis.[21]

Type of burn

There is little evidence that the mechanism of burning injury affects subsequent prognosis, provided that other factors, such as percentage of deep burn and respiratory injury are held constant. Flame and gasoline burns justifiably have a bad reputation, but this is attributable to the severity of the injury rather than any intrinsic feature of the source of heat.

Respiratory injury

Inhalation injury or direct thermal damage to the respiratory lining confers a reduced prognosis to the burned patient. With improvements in the control of infection pulmonary complications have surpassed sepsis as the major cause of death in some centres. Statistical analysis of the effects

mortality and accounted for 68% of deaths in those over 70 years of age. Many deaths in the elderly population of burned patients are due to pre-existing disease as discussed above.

The advances that have taken place in reducing mortality in recent years are a result of improvements in the management of many of these complications. Early wound excision and closure is a good example of a successful attempt to reduce the incidence of wound sepsis. As a by-product of these efforts, in-patient stay has been reduced in some series,[24,31] and length of survival in those eventually succumbing has been extended.[2]

The prediction of mortality

The question of whether a particular burn injury will cause death in a given patient is one which has grasped the attention of many burn specialists. These have attempted from their own accumulated experience to produce statistically derived models, charts or formulae which when applied to the context under consideration will give an accurate prediction. It may be of value to consider the possible applications of these risk models.

Applications

1. To predict the outcome in a particular patient.[2,7,23,34] Predictions on an individual basis must be made with caution, bearing in mind that the characteristics of the patient and his injury are unique, and his response to treatment may be atypical. Indeed, the decision to actively treat or not, when presented with a patient whose prognosis on the indices is very poor, must not be made solely on a prediction.
2. As an aid in patient management.[7,16,23,34] This refers mainly to the concept of triage; patients may be divided into risk categories for referral or transfer to the appropriate unit.
3. As a means of describing and defining a given population of burned patients, in terms of severity.[15,16,35]
4. For review and audit of a series.[2,16,17] The aim is to study the reasons for individual variance from the prognosis prediction, in order to improve management or uncover possible causes of unexpected survival.

Table 13.1. *Lethal area of burn for 50% of the population (SE), by age and time period*

Age	1965–1971	1972–1975	1976–1979
0–4	51.1(2.3)	57.8(3.0)	60.0(4.2)
5–34	61.2(1.4)	68.4(1.8)	71.2(2.3)
35–49	49.7(2.0)	54.5(2.3)	61.8(3.1)
50–59	42.8(2.5)	45.0(2.5)	52.1(3.2)
60–74	27.4(2.0)	33.2(2.0)	33.7(2.3)
>75	16.8(2.8)	18.5(1.9)	19.6(1.9)
Total	52.0(0.9)	56.8(1.1)	59.1(1.4)

Source: From Feller, Tholen, and Cornell.[6]

5. For evaluating and comparing institutions.[15,17,23] This has been done with some benefit among the participants of the NBIE.[4,16] Many other authors have compared the performance of their units with Bull's original grids, derived from the experience of the Birmingham burns unit.[1–3]

6. For the assessment of new techniques or therapies.[2,12,16,18]

7. To assist in the counselling of patients and their families.[16,36] Imbus and Zawacki[37] have presented a sensitive approach to the patient with a hopeless prognosis.

Statistical approaches

It is beyond the scope of this chapter to provide a detailed commentary on the various statistical methods that have been employed in the analysis of severity factors, and in the setting up of mortality prediction models. However, a brief review is in order. The development of patient injury severity indices, not only in burns therapy but in any field, dates back to Bull and Squire in 1949.[1] For a large group of burn patients they plotted the mortality against the area of burn for different age groups and obtained a series of sigmoid curves. By probit transformation these were converted into linear form and a probit formula for each slope was derived. From these formulae the LA50 for each age group could be calculated. The LA50 can be conveniently used for comparing survival statistics between series, either chronologically in the same unit to assess progress or between units to compare performance. An example of the use of LA50 in chronological studies is given in Table 13.1, from data collected in the NBIE survey.[6]

A drawback of probit analysis is that a significant proportion of patients die with other clearly identifiable severity factors, such as smoke inhalation or unusually large full thickness burn areas. Multivariate analytical methods such as multifactorial probit,[18] discriminant function[17] and logistic regression[21] analyses attempt to relate the role of several such severity factors to the outcome. In general, these are more valuable as retrospective surveys in a single unit or group of units than is the comparison of different centres' performance.

The variables selected for inclusion in the analyses necessarily depend on the views and experience of the analysts. There are many published studies which include a selection of the severity factors discussed above. Because the experience of each unit varies, different authors will place emphasis on different variables and this is one reason why this type of analysis is less valuable as an inter-unit assessment. Multivariate methods are, however, particularly useful tools in the audit of improvements in burn care and in assessing the relative roles of the various severity factors in mortality. Particularly useful reviews of statistical analytical methods in burn mortality have been made by Margosches[38] and Bowser.[36]

Indices and scoring systems

There are a number of potentially valuable but complex mortality probability formulae and equations.[16,23] However, there is a distinct role for the simple scoring system or chart which may be used in the emergency department or admission room as a rule-of-thumb assessment of the burn patient, and later when auditing outcome on an individual or series basis. The following may be found useful:

The Bull grid (Fig. 13.1)

From the probit analysis of their data in 1949 Bull and Squire[1] produced a mortality grid. This relates the mortality probability (in decimals) for groups of patients with any combination of age and %TBSA burned. This was updated in 1954,[2] and finally in 1971,[3] and the latter is reproduced in the figure. It must be stressed that the advances in burn care and survival since 1971 mean that the probability figures are likely to tend towards the pessimistic, and that the grid is not a final arbiter for the individual patient. It is much more appropriate as a guide to performance in a burn unit, when individual probabilities are summated and the total compared with the mortality figure for the group.

Body area burned (%)	Age (years)																
	0–4	5–9	10–14	15–19	20–24	25–29	30–34	35–39	40–44	45–49	50–54	55–59	60–64	65–69	70–74	75–79	80+
93+	1	1	1	1	1	1	1	1	1	1	1	1	1	1	1	1	1
88–92	·9	·9	·9	·9	1	1	1	1	1	1	1	1	1	1	1	1	1
83–87	·9	·9	·9	·9	·9	·9	1	1	1	1	1	1	1	1	1	1	1
78–82	·8	·8	·8	·8	·9	·9	·9	·9	1	1	1	1	1	1	1	1	1
73–77	·7	·7	·8	·8	·8	·8	·9	·9	·9	1	1	1	1	1	1	1	1
68–72	·6	·6	·7	·7	·7	·8	·8	·8	·9	·9	·9	1	1	1	1	1	1
63–67	·5	·5	·6	·6	·6	·7	·7	·8	·8	·9	·9	1	1	1	1	1	1
58–62	·4	·4	·4	·5	·5	·6	·6	·7	·7	·8	·9	·9	1	1	1	1	1
53–57	·3	·3	·3	·4	·4	·5	·5	·6	·7	·7	·8	·9	1	1	1	1	1
48–52	·2	·2	·3	·3	·3	·3	·4	·5	·6	·6	·7	·8	·9	1	1	1	1
43–47	·2	·2	·2	·2	·2	·3	·3	·4	·4	·5	·6	·7	·8	1	1	1	1
38–42	·1	·1	·1	·1	·2	·2	·2	·3	·3	·4	·5	·6	·8	·9	1	1	1
33–37	·1	·1	·1	·1	·1	·1	·2	·2	·3	·3	·4	·5	·7	·8	·9	1	1
28–32	0	0	0	0	·1	·1	·1	·1	·2	·2	·3	·4	·6	·7	·9	1	1
23–27	0	0	0	0	0	0	·1	·1	·1	·2	·2	·3	·4	·6	·7	·9	1
18–22	0	0	0	0	0	0	0	·1	·1	·1	·1	·2	·3	·4	·6	·8	·9
13–17	0	0	0	0	0	0	0	0	0	·1	·1	·1	·2	·3	·5	·6	·7
8–12	0	0	0	0	0	0	0	0	0	0	·1	·1	·1	·2	·3	·5	·5
3–7	0	0	0	0	0	0	0	0	0	0	0	0	·1	·1	·2	·3	·4
0–2	0	0	0	0	0	0	0	0	0	0	0	0	0	·1	·1	·2	·2

Fig. 13.1. Mortality probability chart (1965–70). (Reproduced, with permission from Bull.[3])

Bull and Fisher[2] introduced a correction factor for the healthy over-55s. From the patient's age, half the number of years in excess of 55 is subtracted and the table entered at this value instead of the actual age of the patient.

The Baux index[20,34]

This was originally proposed in a thesis by Baux in 1961. It is widely used as a simple working guide. The age of the patient is added to the %TBSA burned. As originally suggested, a value of more than 75 indicates an almost certain probability of death. Due to improved survival, Stern and Waisbren[39] have modified the index by excluding patients under 20 years of age, and stating that the patient has a greater than 50% chance of death if the sum of age and %TBSA burn is more than 95. They found the index performed well in comparison with probit and multifactorial analyses.

The Roi nomogram (Fig. 13.2)

Roi and colleagues produced this graphical method for estimating mortality risk on admission.[7] It requires only the age of the patient, the %TBSA burned, and the knowledge of the presence or absence of a perineal burn. It is based on NBIE data on 11 200 patients, in 1981,

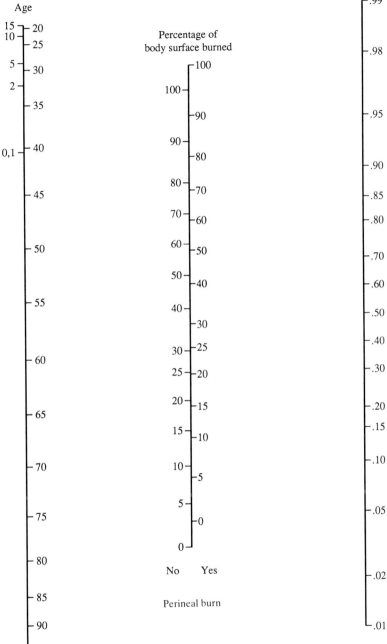

Fig. 13.2. Nomogram for computation of mortality risk for the burned patient. (Reproduced, with permission from Roi *et al.*[7])

Table 13.2. *Abbreviated burn severity index*

Variable	Patient characteristic	Score
Sex	Female	1
	Male	0
Age in years	0–20	1
	21–40	2
	41–60	3
	61–80	4
	81–100	5
Inhalation injury	Present	1
Full thickness burn	Present	1
%TBSA burned	1–10	1
	11–20	2
	21–30	3
	31–40	4
	41–50	5
	51–60	6
	61–70	7
	71–80	8
	81–90	9
	91–100	10

Total burn score	Threat to life	Probability of survival (%)
2–3	Very low	>99
4–5	Moderate	98
6–7	Moderately severe	80–90
8–9	Serious	50–70
10–11	Severe	20–40
12–13	Maximum	<10

Source: Reproduced, with permission, from Tobiasen *et al.*[22]

simplified from a multiple logistic model. A ruler is placed between the relevant points on the two scales of severity factors and the mortality risk read off where the straight edge cuts the risk line.

Tobiasen's abbreviated burn severity index (Table 13.2)

In an attempt to produce a simple but accurate index that reflected other important factors as well as age and %TBSA burn, Tobiasen and colleagues[22] produced a scoring system based on multivariate logistic regression analysis on 590 patients. The presence of an inhalation injury was assumed when two or more criteria were met. These criteria are a) a fire in an enclosed space, b) facial burns with singed nasal hair, c) carbonaceous sputum, and d) stridor or dyspnoea. The other variables are sex and presence or absence of full thickness burn. The total score is equated to a probability of survival scale.

Trends in survival

Over the past three decades a steady increase in LA_{50} values has been apparent. This has been seen in all age groups, although numbers in the group of massive burns over the age of 50 are small and make improvements difficult to detect. These improvements are best documented in the reports from the NBIE (Table 13.1), in which analysis suggests that early excision as a policy has been largely responsible for the improvements. It must be acknowledged that a raised level of interest and commitment due to the data collection initiatives must also play a significant part. Among children, reported improvements in survival have been so dramatic that in some centres children might be expected to survive almost any burn, provided that there is no serious respiratory injury.[11]

Marked advances in prognosis have been attributed to other factors entirely, in a report from Liljedahl and colleagues.[40] They use exposure management of the burn in warm dry air which minimizes heat loss and metabolic requirements. Deep burns are not excised early but covered with homograft or heterograft after informal debridement. Again, the experience and enthusiasm of the burn team is crucial.

Improvements in prognosis of the burned patient will continue as long as the energy of dedicated burn team members continues to be applied to the problems remaining; the prediction of survival when appropriately applied is a valuable aid in this endeavour.

References

1 Bull JP, Squire JR. A study of mortality in a burns unit. *Ann Surg* 1949; **130**:160.
2 Bull JP, Fisher AJ. A study of mortality in a burns unit: a revised estimate. *Ann Surg* 1954; **139**:269.
3 Bull JP. Revised analysis of mortality due to burns. *Lancet* 1971; **ii**:1133.
4 Feller I, Flora JD, Bawol R. Baseline results of therapy for burned patients. *J Am Med Assn* 1976; **236**:1943.
5 Cornell RG, Feller I, Roi LD *et al.* Evaluation of burn care utilizing a national burn registry. *Emerg Med Serv* 1978; **7**:107.

6 Feller I, Tholen D, Cornell RG. Improvements in burn care, 1965–1979. *J Am Med Assn* 1980; **244**:2074.

7 Roi LD, Flora JD, Davis TM *et al.* A severity grading chart for the burned patient. *Ann Emerg Med* 1981; **10**:161.

8 Wolfe RA, Roi LD, Flora JD *et al.* Mortality differences and speed of wound closure among specialized burn care facilities. *J Am Med Assn* 1983; **250**:763.

9 Demling RH. Improved survival after massive burns. *J Trauma* 1983; **23**:179.

10 Tompkins RG, Burke JF, Schoenfeld DA *et al.* Prompt eschar excision: a treatment system contributing to reduced burn mortality. *Ann Surg* 1986; **204**:272.

11 Herndon DN, Le Marter J, Beard S *et al.* The quality of life after major thermal injury in children. *J Trauma* 1986; **26**:609.

12 Feller I, Jones CA. The National Burn Information Exchange. The use of a National Burn Registry to evaluate and address the burn problem. *Surg Clin N Am* 1987; **67**:167.

13 Pruitt BA, Tumbusch WT, Mason AD, Pearson E. Mortality in 110 consecutive burns treated at a Burns Unit. *Ann Surg* 1964; **159**:396.

14 Rittenbury MS, Maddox RW, Schmidt FH *et al.* Probit analysis of burn mortality in 1831 patients: comparison with other large series. *Ann Surg* 1966; **164**:123.

15 McCoy JA, Micks DW, Lynch JB. Discriminant function probability model for predicting survival in burned patients. *J Am Med Assn* 1968; **203**:128.

16 Roi LD, Flora JD, Davis TM, Wolfe RA. Two new burn severity indices. *J Trauma* 1983; **23**:1023.

17 Moores B, Rahman MM, Browning FSC, Settle JAD. Discriminant function analysis of 570 consecutive burn patients admitted to the Yorkshire Regional Burns Centre between 1966 and 1973. *Burns* 1975; **1**:135.

18 Zawacki BE, Azen SP, Imbus SH *et al.* Multifactorial probit analysis of mortality in burned patients. *Ann Surg* 1979; **189**:1.

19 Barrow RE, Herndon DN. Incidence of mortality in boys and girls after severe thermal burns. *Surg Gyn Obst* 1990; **170**:295.

20 Baux S, Mimoun M, Saade H *et al.* Burns in the elderly. *Burns* 1989; **15**:239.

21 Berry CC, Wachtel TL, Frank HA. An analysis of factors which predict mortality in hospitalized burn patients. *Burns* 1982; **9**:38.

22 Tobiasen J, Hiebert JM, Edlich RF. The abbreviated burn severity index. *Ann Emerg Med* 1982; **11**:260.

23 Clark CJ, Reid WH, Gilmour WH, Campbell D. Mortality probability in victims of fire trauma: revised equation to include inhalation injury. *Br Med J* 1986; **292**:1303.

24 Deitch EA. A policy of early excision and grafting in elderly burn patients shortens the hospital stay and improves survival. *Burns* 1985; **12**:109.

25 Herndon DN, Gore D, Cole M *et al.* Determinants of mortality in paediatric patients with greater than 70% full thickness total body surface area thermal injury treated by early total excision and grafting. *J Trauma* 1987; **27**:208.

26 Tompkins RG, Remensnyder JP, Burke JF *et al.* Significant reductions in mortality for children with burn injuries through the use of prompt eschar excision. *Ann Surg* 1988; **208**:577.

27 Tompkins RG, Hilton JF, Burke JF *et al.* Increased survival after massive thermal injuries in adults: Preliminary report using artificial skin. *Crit Care Med* 1989; **17**:734.

28 Yarbrough DR. Improving survival in the burned patient. *J S Carolina Med Assoc* 1990; **86(6)**:347.

29 Manson WL, Westerveld AW, Klasen HJ *et al.* Selective intestinal decontamination of the digestive tract for infection prophylaxis in severely burned patients. *Scand J Plast Reconstr Surg* 1987; **21**:269.

30 Herndon DN, Barrow RE, Stein M *et al.* Increased mortality with intravenous supplemental feeding in severely burned patients. *J Burn Care & Rehabil* 1989; **10**:309.

31 Curreri PW, Luterman A, Braun DW *et al.* Burn injury analysis of survival and hospitalization time for 937 patients. *Ann Surg* 1980; **192**:472.

32 Achauer BM, Allyn PA, Furnas DW *et al.* Pulmonary complications of burns: the major threat to the burn patient. *Ann Surg* 1973; **177**:311.

33 Le HQ, Zamboni W, Eriksson E *et al.* Burns in patients under two and over 70 years of age. *Ann Plast Surg* 1986; **17**:39.

34 Tobiasen J, Hiebert JH, Edlich RF. Prediction of burn mortality. *Surg Gynecol Obstet* 1982; **154**:711.

35 Fisher J, Wells JA, Fulwinder BT *et al.* Editorial: Do we need a burn severity grading system? *J Trauma* 1977; 17:252.

36 Bowser BH, Caldwell FT, Baker JA *et al.* Statistical methods to predict morbidity and mortality: self assessment techniques for burn units. *Burns* 1983; **9**:318.

37 Imbus SH, Zawacki BE. Autonomy for burned patients when survival is unprecedented. *N Eng J Med* 1977; **297**:308.

38 Margosches EH, Roi LD, Flora JD. The statistical analysis of burn patient data: a historical review. *Burns* 1978; **5**:43.

39 Stern M, Waisbren BA. Comparison of methods of predicting burn mortality. *Burns* 1979; **6**:119.

40 Liljedahl SO, Lamke LO, Jonsson CE *et al.* Warm dry air treatment of 345 patients with burns exceeding 20 per cent of the body surface. *Scand J Plast Reconstr Surg* 1979; **13**:205.

14

Complications of intensive care of the burned patient

S.M. UNDERWOOD, L.T.A. RYLAH

Introduction

A major burn injury poses a threat to life which necessitates intensive nursing and medical care. Complications may develop and these will be dealt with in respect to their relevant systems in this chapter.

Respiratory

The incidence of pulmonary complications associated with burn injury is approximately 22% but the mortality of this group is of the order of 80%.[1] Early complications result from upper airway obstruction by oedema, which may go on developing for up to 48 hours, bronchospasm and inhalation of toxic vapours.

Intubation to secure the airway must be considered early as it will become more difficult as oedema develops. Tracheostomy is avoided as it is associated with an increased mortality if performed as an emergency. A serious complication of nasal intubation is sinus infection[2] but the security of fixation of the tube, which may be impossible to replace in the first few days, is so important that the nasal route is preferable to oral intubation. If the tube cannot be satisfactorily taped in position, it must be sutured in place. Oral tubes may be sutured to the teeth.

Fluid resuscitation must not be decreased, but rather increased if inhalational injury accompanies a cutaneous burn since it will improve circulatory support without worsening lung oedema.[3] Steroid therapy is no longer advocated as it has been shown to be associated with an increased infection rate and mortality.[4] Prophylactic antibiotics are not recommended as their use results in infection by resistant bacteria. Sputum must be cultured regularly and if infection develops appropriate antibiotic therapy must be instituted.

188

As airway oedema subsides, over the 3–4 days after the injury, increased mucus production along with reduction in cilial activity combine to increase the risk of infection. Debris becomes detached from the small airways, which then become obstructed, and thus will add to the increased shunt fraction seen following major burns. The application of positive end expiratory pressure (PEEP) or continuous positive airway pressure (CPAP) helps to keep small airways patent, reducing collapse and hypoxia as long as cardiac output is not compromised. Positive pressure is also useful in treating pulmonary oedema due to inhalational injury. Inspired gases must be warmed and humidified to reduce heat loss and decrease sputum tenacity. Physiotherapy is of utmost importance at this stage if pneumonia is to be avoided. Wheezing is treated with nebulized bronchodilators such as salbutamol.

Controlled, usually intermittent positive pressure ventilation (IPPV), is frequently necessary for patients with major burn injury particularly if there is an accompanying inhalational injury. Adult respiratory distress syndrome (ARDS) is well described in association with major burn injury, possibly due to mediators released from the burn or resulting from inhalational injury damaging the pulmonary capillary–endothelial membrane. Debridement of the burn wound results in a temporary decrease in lung function, possibly secondary to release of endotoxin or other mediators from the burn area. Major burn injury is followed by a rise in metabolic rate. Failure to comprehend this and provide sufficient minute volume ventilation will result in hypercarbia.

Any severely ill patient on the intensive care unit may succumb to complications arising from mechanical ventilation. However, mechanical ventilation with the use of muscle relaxation and adequate sedation will decrease the work of breathing, and thus decrease the oxygen demand, by up to 25% in a septic patient. This will allow better use of the available oxygen. Muscle relaxation and sedation in a balanced technique will also allow the cardiovascular system to be adequately monitored and manipulated, if this is necessary. Higher inspired oxygen concentrations and faster rates of breathing will allow the blood gas chemistry to be optimized. The benefit of these procedures has to be weighed against the additional risks involved in these techniques.

The size of tracheal tube used must be chosen carefully to avoid complications arising from prolonged intubation. Tracheal stenosis can result from burn injury or as a complication of the trauma produced by prolonged intubation. Modern plastic tubes with low-pressure, high-volume cuffs reduce this risk but cases of sub-glottic stenosis have been

reported, particularly in association with inhalational injury.[5] Pneumothorax is more likely if high inflation pressures are required due to lung
damage by toxic inhalation or as ARDS develops.

Circumferential burns cause constriction of the chest which makes
breathing difficult and requires high inflation pressures on IPPV. This is
improved with escharotomy which will be required as an emergency
procedure on the intensive care unit.

Patients with major burns have many of the risk factors associated with
thromboembolic phenomena: they require multiple vascular cannula-
tions, undergo multiple operations, are immobile for long periods and
suffer massive fluid shifts. In children the incidence of fatal pulmonary
embolism following burn injury is 1.7%.[6] The incidence of clinically
diagnosed pulmonary embolism in adults is 0.4%[7] so prophylactic hepari-
nization is not recommended except in obesity, those with burns of less
than 15% of the lower limbs and those with a history of thrombo-embolic
disease. The increased risk of gastro-intestinal bleeding associated with
larger burns precludes the use of anti-coagulants in patients with major
burn injury.

Cardiovascular

The commonest cardiovascular problem on the intensive care unit is
hypovolaemia. This is avoided by careful fluid replacement according to
one of the formulae used for resuscitation (Chapter 4) but remembering
that each patient is different and that adjustments to the regime may be
necessary, particularly in small children, the elderly and those with
concurrent underlying pathology. Adjustments can often be decided by
the clinical condition of the patient but occasionally require more
invasive monitoring.

Central venous cannulation is avoided if at all possible in the burn
patient because of the high infection risk. Other complications are similar
to those in other patients, namely bleeding, haematoma, pneumothorax,
haemothorax, nerve damage, dysrhythmias, air or catheter embolus and
thrombosis.

A pulmonary artery catheter will be useful for monitoring and manipulation of cardiovascular parameters in the severely ill patient. It must be
ensured that the advantages it confers outweigh the risks, particularly
that of infection. Other complications include those of central venous
cannulation as well as perforation of the pulmonary artery, pulmonary
infarction and injury to the pulmonary or tricuspid valves, although these

are infrequent.[8] All central venous catheters must be removed at the earliest possible time to avoid complications.

In the first few hours after a major burn injury the myocardium is depressed by factors released into the plasma[9] and the vasculature loses its integrity. Inotropes may be necessary to support the circulation until vascular integrity returns and myocardial depression wanes at about 6–12 hours. Inotropic support may be required at this time and is associated with complications of its own; both those of central line insertion and the adverse effects of the drugs used. Catecholamines produce tachycardia and dysrhythmias and some have vasodilator action which can result in hypotension making a combination of drugs preferable. As a hypermetabolic state supervenes the circulation becomes hyperdynamic, and cardiac output and oxygen consumption are increased. If coronary blood flow is limited by coronary artery disease, it cannot increase to supply sufficient oxygen to meet the increased needs of the myocardium, which will become ischaemic.

Irreversible burn shock occurs in a few patients who fail to respond to fluid resuscitation; it is almost invariably fatal. Plasma exchange has been used in some such patients on the assumption that circulating serum factors are responsible.[10] Improvement in fluid requirements, urine output and lactic acidosis has been seen after plasma exchange.

Heart failure occurs if fluid replacement is overzealous in patients with little cardiac reserve or in those who develop myocardial ischaemia. It may also occur later if oedema fluid resorption is rapid. It is treated by reducing the sodium load and supporting the myocardium with positive inotropes. Diuretics may be given but will cloud the response to resuscitation.

Dysrhythmias are a complication of electrical burns but also occur with hypokalaemia and other electrolyte disturbances which can result from rapid fluid replacement. Continuous electrocardiographic monitoring alerts the physician to any dysrhythmia, which can be treated appropriately, usually by correcting the electrolyte imbalance but occasionally with anti-dysrhythmic agents. Patients admitted with electrical burns will need 24-hour ECG monitoring. However, after the initial insult, dysrhythmias are unlikely. Sequelae usually occur if myocardial damage has been produced by a period of hypoxaemia due to cardiac arrest or ventricular fibrillation.

Systemic arterial hypertension occurs if the raised cardiac output enters a noncompliant vasculature, for example in patients with arteriosclerosis. It occurs in children, the highest risk group being males aged

7–10 years and burns over 20% in whom the incidence is 57%.[11] If untreated, it is associated with increased morbidity in the form of encephalopathic complications resulting in seizures, but not in increased mortality. It subsides when the burn area is healed.

Circumferential burns may compromise blood supply in limbs and require urgent escharotomy.

Endocarditis is a later complication which results from infected catheters, particularly those placed in central vessels. Treatment includes removal of old lines and replacement, if necessary, with new ones along with antibiotic therapy appropriate to the offending organism.

Endocrine

Burn injury is associated with a marked endocrine response.[12] Catecholamines and cortisol are raised and impaired glucose tolerance is a common feature. Insulin infusion may be required but blood sugar must be measured regularly, particularly in the sedated patient, in whom dangerous hypoglycaemia is difficult to recognize clinically, and in children, in whom it is more common. Large amounts of insulin may be needed as this form of hyperglycaemia is very insulin resistant.

Immune function is suppressed more in burned than other trauma patients, rendering them highly susceptible to infection. Various immune suppressive factors have been isolated from burn serum; they may originate from burn tissue or be released by an intense local inflammatory response following severe burn injury.[13] Burn patients are also subject to other factors which decrease immune response, namely repeated anaesthesia and surgery, blood transfusion, various drugs, malnutritional states and the stress response to major injury.

Endotoxin, released from macrophages, elicits the production of tumour necrosis factor (TNF) which causes coagulopathy, shock, fluid and electrolyte sequestration, widespread organ damage and is in itself a pyrogen. The resetting of the hypothalamic thermostat to make the patient pyrexial, usually 38–39 °C, decreases the role of temperature in the clinical diagnosis of infection. TNF also stimulates interleukin–1 production by phagocytic cells which mediates the acute phase response, including the immunological changes. Serum TNF levels are highest in association with bouts of infection and in those patients who ultimately succumb to burn injury.[14]

Adrenal insufficiency occurs in some patients with severe shock due to hypovolaemia or sepsis, and must be suspected in patients not responding normally to resuscitation. Replacement therapy will have a dramatic effect.

Haematology

Both hyper-coagulability and hypo-coagulability are seen in the patient who has sustained a major burn. Initial fluid shifts result in a high haematocrit which is later reduced by effective fluid resuscitation. Early anaemia is the result of thermal damage to red blood cells but later it is more likely to result from repeated operations, gastrointestinal bleeding, bone marrow suppression due to infection, decreased erythropoiesis or even repeated blood sampling.[15] Transfusion may be necessary to keep the haematocrit above 0.3 and ensure adequate oxygen transport.

Both the cellular and the humoral arms of the body's defence system are less effective following a burn injury than usual. White cell count will be raised following burn injury but function is poor, reducing resistance to infection. Granulocyte colony-stimulating factor has been given to mice and in association with antibiotic therapy showed an increased survival rate after burn injury;[16] it may prove useful in man in the future. Leucopaenia has been associated with topical silver sulphadiazine therapy and appears to be self-limiting.[17]

Large burns are managed best by early excision and grafting which is a major blood-losing operation. Massive blood transfusions are necessary to maintain haemodynamic stability. The usual complications arise; hypothermia, avoided by use of a blood warmer, citrate intoxication and potassium shifts. Coagulopathy is improved by administration of fresh frozen plasma as soon as surgery is complete and platelet transfusion if the count is low and there is active bleeding.

Gastrointestinal tract

Paralytic ileus occurs several days after burn injury. It may be associated with electrolyte imbalance, particularly hypokalaemia, and is also a sign of underlying sepsis. Insertion of a nasogastric tube reduces the distension as well as discomfort to the patient. Gastric perforation is more likely with larger burns and can occur some days after injury.

Superior mesenteric artery syndrome (SMAS) occurs about a month after injury, usually when there has been significant weight loss. Bilious vomiting is accompanied by early satiety and post-prandial abdominal fullness which may be relieved by limiting oral intake or changing position. In a large group of patients, with mean burn area of 34%, 1% developed SMAS.[18] The duodenum becomes obstructed by the superior mesenteric artery. Initial treatment consists of lying the patient prone, nasogastric decompression, administration of intravenous fluids and hyperalimentation. Some patients require operation, most commonly duodeno-jejunostomy.

Aetiological factors suggested in acalculus cholecystitis in the burn patient include dehydration, prolonged ileus, sepsis, blood transfusion, SMAS and decreased tissue oxygenation.[19] Diagnosis may be aided by ultrasound, but early surgery for the acute abdomen may be life-saving.

Pancreatitis may also occur in the burned patient on the intensive care unit. It may result from hypoperfusion, vascular changes, decreased gut motility or be part of the sepsis syndrome. Severe complications may ensue; ARDS, renal or hepatic failure and disseminated intravascular coagulation among them.[20] A high serum amylase will be diagnostic and surgical intervention contra-indicated.

Gastric and duodenal ulceration occurs in over 20% of burned patients. Antacids and H_2 antagonists reduce the incidence of bleeding and are often given prophylactically to patients with major burns. Ranitidine at 0.125 mg per kilogram per hour by infusion up to a total dose of 3 mg per kg per day will avoid high bolus levels, and has been used with success on children in the authors' unit. Early enteral nutrition also reduces gastrointestinal bleeding.[21] When preventive measures are not utilized, or fail, and massive haemorrhage or perforation occur, gastric resection is required.[22]

There is some concern that raising gastric pH increases the likelihood of bacteraemia and septicaemia as the gut flora is altered and defence mechanisms reduced. Sucralfate, an aluminium salt of sucrose, provides protection against stress bleeding without affecting gastric pH thereby reducing the incidence of nosocomial pneumonia when compared with antacid therapy.[23] Selective decontamination of the gastrointestinal tract is another solution to this problem.[24] However, widespread use of antibiotics results in resistant strains of bacteria which are a problem in the burn unit where infection is already a major cause of death. Antibiotic therapy is not without hazard; pseudomembranous colitis is a serious complication, and must be treated with vancomycin, and cardiovascular and respiratory support if severe.

Liver dysfunction occurs in as many as 58% of burned patients, the highest incidence being in those with the largest burned areas.[25] Early liver damage appears to be related to the severity of cardiovascular instability and can occur 24 hours after the burn. Hepatocellular injury results in raised transaminases, alkaline phosphatase and bilirubin. Jaundice is associated with increased mortality. A non-specific hepatitic picture emerges later with intrahepatic cholestasis in septic patients accentuated by blood transfusion or haemolysis. Treatment consists of maintaining liver blood supply and providing early wound cover.

Renal, fluid and electrolytes

During the resuscitation phase patients with burns over 15% in adults, or 10% in children, require urinary catheterization. Scrupulous aseptic technique is required for insertion since bacteria introduced at this stage can easily result in sepsis.

Inadequate fluid resuscitation results in decreased renal blood flow and the possibility of acute tubular necrosis. If haemoglobinuria accompanies hypovolaemia, the risk of renal failure is increased (*vide infra*). Prevention of hypovolaemia and maintenance of urine output reduce this risk.

During initial resuscitation, intravenous fluids containing sodium and water are administered. Later, sodium is only necessary for maintenance and dextrose is added as glycogen stores are reduced. Electrolyte imbalance can occur in the immediate resuscitation period as large volumes of fluid are given, or later if parenteral nutrition is required or gastro-intestinal complications supervene. If fluid is lost into the gut, hyponatraemia and hypokalaemia are seen. Gastric dilation is associated with hypochloraemic alkalosis. Massive blood transfusion is associated with transient hypocalcaemia and potassium shifts.

Hypocalcaemia and hypermagnesaemia are consequences of major burn injury.[26] The fact that total protein is low makes a low total calcium unsurprising, but ionized calcium is also reduced, at least for the first week after injury, even if adequate replacement is given. Calcium is involved in muscle contraction, including that of the myocardium and peripheral vasculature. Infusion of calcium can cause cardiac dysrhythmias and if required must be given during electrocardiographic monitoring.

Hypophosphataemia is a feature of major burn injury.[27] One cause is reduced phosphate uptake from the gut as a result of aluminium hydroxide antacid therapy. Others are loss of phosphate from burned skin, starvation and parenteral nutrition. Hypophosphataemia is important since patients with the lowest phosphate levels have the highest mortality. It results in dysfunction of red cells, leucocytes, platelets and brain cells.

Table 14.1. *Ideal urine output during fluid resuscitation (mg/kg/h)*

	Pigmenturia	
	Not present	Present
Adults	0.5–0.7	1.5
Children (<30 kg)	1	3
Infants (<10 kg)	2	5–6

Cells become deficient in ATP and oxygen delivery from haemoglobin is decreased via a reduction in 2,3-diphosphoglycerate.

Trace elements and minerals become depleted in the intensive care patient, particularly when parenteral nutrition is necessary or diet is inadequate. Zinc has been shown to influence healing. Trace elements, minerals and vitamins can be added to the diet but the establishment of a full balanced diet as early as possible is the best treatment.

Pigmenturia

The presence of large amounts of haemochromogens in the urine may complicate high-voltage electrical burns or extensive deep thermal injuries during the immediate post-burn period. The amount of haemochromogens appears to be directly related to the volume of muscle injured. It is also seen with other severe muscle injury resulting in necrosis[28] and crush injuries. The passage of darkly pigmented urine (burgundy-brown) is the most reliable clinical sign and must elicit a prompt and aggressive therapeutic response from the clinician. The rate of fluid administration must be increased to achieve a minimum urine flow rate of 1.5 ml per kilogram per hour in adults or up to twice this in children under 30 kg (Table 14.1). The immediate infusion of 12.5 grams of mannitol in a 20% or 25% solution as an intravenous bolus in an adult will help to initiate urine flow. As myoglobin is less likely to precipitate in an alkaline urine approximately 1 mmol per kilogram of sodium bicarbonate is added to each litre of resuscitation fluid until the serum pH, and thus urinary pH is alkaline. Once all gross pigment is cleared from the urine, the resuscitation fluid is decreased once more to obtain a urine output of 0.5 ml per kilogram per hour. Hourly urine samples are collected and compared to monitor this progressive change in colour.

Neurological and musculoskeletal

Electrical burns are associated with some neurological sequelae. About half of the low voltage injuries in one series[29] were followed by neurological symptoms although most resolved. Immediate unconsciousness is associated with high voltage injury (45%) and is of variable duration with a poorer prognosis for those still unconscious on admission to hospital. If the victim survives and hypoxia has been avoided, sequelae are uncommon. Initial paralysis may be transient. The peripheral neuropathies seen after high voltage injury recover more often (64%) than those of delayed onset.

Neuropathy can develop in patients who spend a long time on the intensive care unit. Deficiency of trace elements may be a factor but a neuropathy of long-term immobilization appears to exist which is most disabling as the patient improves and attempts to mobilize. It may result in prolongation of the requirement for mechanical ventilation and usually recovers slowly. Peripheral neuropathy has been demonstrated in 29% of patients with burns over 20%. In a third of the patients studied, proximal myopathy was also seen but was thought to be due to repeated intramuscular injections.[30]

Burn patients exhibit electromyographic changes similar to those of denervation or myopathy.[31] It is well known that administration of the depolarising muscle relaxant succinylcholine more than two days after injury may result in potentially fatal hyperkalaemia in the burn patient.[32] The patient with a major burn may require 2.5 to 5 times the usual dose of a non-depolarizing muscle relaxant. Resistance peaks about two weeks after the burn then decreases as the wound heals although it can persist for some time after complete wound healing.[33] If a site is available, neuromuscular monitoring will be helpful when relaxation is required for artificial ventilation or during operative procedures. Reversal of neuromuscular blockade is effected with the usual doses of antagonist drugs, if these are necessary.

Myopathy is also seen in long-term intensive care patients. It may be related to malnutrition or disuse of muscle during immobilization. Contractures and joint deformity occur readily in the immobile patient and their prevention by regular physiotherapy must start early and continue throughout the intensive care unit stay and beyond to maintain mobility.

Toxic shock syndrome carries a mortality of about 11% which is reduced by early recognition and treatment. It is caused by toxin-producing staphlococci and was originally described in menstruating women in association with tampon use. It has now been described in children and in burned patients.[34] It is diagnosed clinically by the presence of fever, rash, hypotension, myalgia, vomiting or diarrhoea, mucous membrane inflammation and laboratory abnormalities of two or more systems with no evidence of other aetiology and may have a rapidly fatal course. Treatment consists of urgent transfusion with fresh frozen plasma at a rate equivalent to the hourly metabolic need for a period of three hours and intravenous antibiotics which must be started immediately on suspicion of the diagnosis.

Pharmacology

If muscle relaxation is used to obtund movement during mechanical ventilation, it will be noticed that much greater doses are needed of all relaxants. The increased basal temperature and hyperdynamic cardiovascular system increase the metabolism and decrease the half-life of these drugs. This is in addition to the resistance that has been noted.

Similarly affected are the opiate analgesics and also other sedative drugs such as propofol, midazolam and lorazepam. Burned patients show a remarkable resistance to their effects.

Plasma levels of antibiotics are affected by the loss from the burn wound, and post-operative bleeding. This must be taken into account when treating life-threatening sepsis. Hypernatraemia may be noticed as some antibiotics will have a significant sodium load when given intravenously.

Nursing

Nursing the patient with a major burn injury provides many challenges. The patient must be nursed in a warm room to avoid excessive heat loss. It must be remembered that the hypothalamic thermostat becomes reset to give the patient a temperature of 38–39 °C which must be regarded as normal and no attempt made at cooling.

In order to allow healing of wound, graft and donor sites low air loss beds are required which minimize pressure on them. Removal of dressings is often painful and requires good analgesia or sometimes general anaesthesia. Analgesia is also important for effective physiotherapy. Opiates are necessary initially and must be given in sufficient doses, even if they produce sedation and respiratory depression necessitating mechanical ventilation.

The patient who has suffered a major burn is at risk of continuing psychological effects which must not be under-estimated since they have a profound effect on physical and mental recovery. The support of the intensive care team can reduce the psychological trauma for the patient.

Summary

Awareness, prevention, early diagnosis and treatment of complications arising in the burned patient on the intensive care unit will ensure a better outcome.

References

1 Achauer BM, Allyn PA, Furnas DW *et al.* Pulmonary complications of burns: the major threat to the burn patient. *Ann Surg* 1973; **177**:311–19.
2 O'Reilly MJ, Reddick EJ, Black W *et al.* Sepsis from sinusitis in nasotracheally intubated patients. *Am J Surg* 1984; **147**:601–4.
3 Herndon DN, Barrow RE, Linares HA *et al.* Inhalational injury in burned patients: effects and treatment. *Burns* 1988; **14**:349–56.
4 Moylan JA, Chan C-K. Inhalational injury – an increasing problem. *Ann Surg* 1978; **188**:34–7.
5 Katalic MR, Burke JF. Severe low pressure cuff tracheal injury in burn patients. *Intens Care Med* 1981; **7**:89–92.
6 Desai MH, Linares HA, Herndon DN. Pulmonary embolism in burned children. *Burns* 1989; **15**:376–80.
7 Purdue GF, Hunt JL. Pulmonary emboli in burned patients. *J Trauma* 1988; **28**:218–20.
8 Elliott CG, Zimmerman GA, Clemmer TP. Complications of pulmonary artery catheterization in the care of critically ill patients. *Chest* 1979; **76**:647–52.
9 Raffa J, Trunkey DD. Myocardial depression in acute thermal injury. *J Trauma* 1978; **18**:90–3.
10 Warden GD, Stratta RJ, Saffle JR *et al.* Plasma exchange therapy in patients failing to resuscitate from burn shock. *J Trauma* 1983; **23**:945–51.
11 Popp MB, Friedberg DL, MacMillan BG. Clinical characteristics of hypertension in burned children. *Ann Surg* 1980; **191**:473–8.
12 Dolecek R. Endocrine changes after burn trauma – a review. *Keio J Med* 1989; **38**:262–76.
13 Hansbrough JF, Zapata-Sirvent R, Hoyt D. Postburn immunosuppression: an inflammatory response to the burn wound? *J Trauma* 1990; **30**:671–5.
14 Marano MA, Fong Y, Moldawer LL *et al.* Serum cachectin/tumour necrosis factor in critically ill patients with burns correlates with infection and mortality. *Surg Gyn Obst* 1990; **170**:32–8.
15 Baar S. Anaemia of burns. *Burns* 1979; **6**:1–8.
16 Silver GM, Gamelli RL, O'Reilly M. The beneficial effect of granulocyte colony-stimulating factor (G-CSF) in combination with gentamicin on survival after Pseudomonas burn wound infection. *Surgery* 1989; **106**:452–6.
17 Jarrett F, Ellerbe S, Demling R. Acute leukopenia during topical burn therapy with silver sulfadiazine. *Am J Surg* 1978; **135**:818–19.
18 Lescher TJ, Sirinek KR, Pruitt BA Jr. Superior mesenteric artery syndrome in thermally injured patients. *J Trauma* 1979; **19**: 567–71.
19 Alawneh I. Acute non-calculus cholecystitis in burns. *Br J Surg* 1978; **65**:243–5.

20 Shinozawa Y, Aikawa N. Complications of burn injury. In: *Acute Management of Burn Trauma.* Martyn JAJ (ed). WB Saunders, Philadelphia, PA, 1990.

21 Moscona R, Kaufman T, Jacobs R *et al.* Prevention of gastrointestinal bleeding in burns: the effects of cimetidine or antacids combined with early enteral nutrition. *Burns* 1985; **12**:65–7.

22 Pruitt BA, Goodwin CW. Stress ulcer disease in the burned patient. *World J Surg* 1981; **5**:209–22.

23 Tryba M. Risk of acute stress bleeding and nosocomial pneumonia in ventilated intensive care unit patients: sucralfate versus antacids. *Am J Med* 1987; **28**:117–24.

24 Ulrich C, Harinck-de Weerd JE, Bakker NC *et al.* Selective decontamination of the digestive tract with norfloxacin in the prevention of ICU-acquired infections: a prospective randomized study. *Intens Care Med* 1989; **15**:424–31.

25 Czaja AJ, Rizzo TA, Smith WR, Pruitt BA. Acute liver disease after cutaneous thermal injury. *J Trauma* 1975; **15**:887–94.

26 Szyfelbein SK, Drop LJ, Martyn JAJ. Persistent ionized hypocalcemia in patients during resuscitation and recovery phases of body burns. *Crit Care Med* 1981; **9**:454–8.

27 Nordstrom H, Lennquist S, Lindell B *et al.* Hypophosphataemia in severe burns. *Acta Chir Scand* 1977; **143**:395–9.

28 Better OS, Stein JH. Current Concepts: early management of shock and prophylaxis of acute renal failure in traumatic rhabdomyolysis. *N Eng J Med* 1990, **322**:825–28.

29 Grube BJ, Heimbach DM, Engrav LH, Copass MK. Neurologic consequences of electric burns. *J Trauma* 1990; **30**:254–8.

30 Helm PA, Johnson ER, Carlton AM. Peripheral neurological problems in the acute burn patient. *Burns* 1976; **3**:123–5.

31 Mills A, Schriefer T, Martyn JAJ. Electromyographic studies of patients with thermal injury. *Anesthesiology* 1986; **65**:A294.

32 Gronert GA, Theye RA. Pathophysiology of hyperkalaemia induced by succinylcholine. *Anesthesiology* 1975; **43**:89–99.

33 Martyn JAJ, Goldhill DR, Goudsouzian NG. Clinical pharmacology of muscle relaxants in patients with burns. *J Clin Pharmacol* 1986; **26**:680–5.

34 Cole RP, Shakespeare PG. Toxic shock syndrome in scalded children. *Burns* 1990; **16**:221–4.

Index

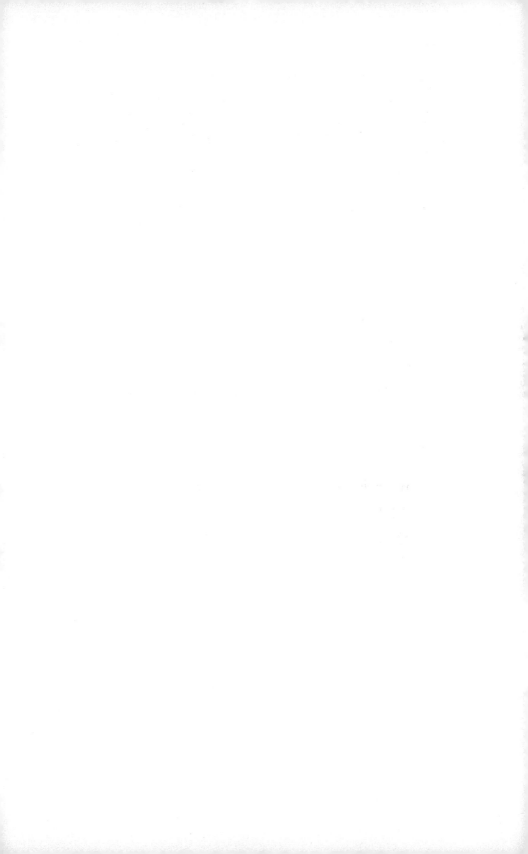